Conceptual Models of Neural Organization

Conceptual Models of Neural Organization

Based on a Work Session
of the Neurosciences Research Program

John Szentágothai and **Michael A. Arbib**

Yvonne Homsy
NRP Writer-Editor

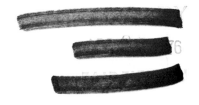

The MIT Press
Cambridge, Massachusetts, and London, England

This book was first published as Volume 12, Number 3, October 1974, of the *Neurosciences Research Program Bulletin*.

The Neurosciences Research Program is sponsored by the Massachusetts Institute of Technology and is supported in part by National Aeronautics and Space Administration, National Institute of Mental Health Grant No. MH23132, National Institute of Neurological Diseases and Stroke Grant No. NS09937, National Science Foundation, Office of Naval Research, The Grant Foundation, Neurosciences Research Foundation, The Rogosin Foundation, and The Alfred P. Sloan Foundation.

First MIT Press edition, 1975. This book was printed and bound in the United States of America.

ISBN: 0-262-19144-X
Library of Congress catalog card number: 75-18837

CONTENTS

Participants viii

I. INTRODUCTION 1

    A Functional Overview 2
    A Structural Overview 3
    Stereopsis 4
    Cerebellar Function 5
    In Retrospect 6

II. A FUNCTIONAL OVERVIEW 7

    General Principles for Adaptive Interaction of a Complex
      System with Its Environment 7
    Principle 1. Theory Must Be Action-Oriented 7
    Principle 2. Perception Is Not Only of "What"
      But Also of "Where" 8
    Principle 3. An Adaptive System Must Be Able to Correlate
      Sensory Data and Actions in Such a Way as to
      Update an Internal Model of the World 8
    Principle 4. Organization Must Be Hierarchical with Adequate
      "Feedback Loops" to Coordinate the Subsystems 10
    Principle 5. The Brain Is a Layered Somatotopic Computer . . . 14
    Multiple Representations 17
      The Somatosensory System 17
      Comparison of Different Sensory Systems 20
      Eye Movements and Visual Perception 23
      Corollary Discharge 27
      Optomotor Behavior in the Fly 29
    Hierarchies of Motor Control 32
      Feedforward and Feedback 33
      Minimal Structural Requirements of Coordinated
      Movement 39
      Complexity and Hierarchies 40

III.   A STRUCTURAL OVERVIEW 42

Neural Networks 42

Neural Network: A Continuum or Separable Units? 44

"Randomness" Versus Specificity of Structure 45

Random or Quasi-Random Neural Networks 50

Significance in Neuron Nets of the General Orientation
of Neuropil Elements 52

The Modular Structure of the Neuropil 58

Stacked Chips of Neuropil 58

Cerebellar Modules 65

Modules of Specific Connectivity 69

Large-Scale Organoid Modules 74

Layer-by-Layer Analysis 76

Organization Principles of Afferent Systems 81

A Comparison of Neuronal and Synaptic Organizations
in the Main Sensory Systems 82

Subcortical Relay Nuclei 85

Organization Principles of Internal Feedback Loops 91

Organization of Large-Scale Feedback Pathways 91

Local Recurrent Couplings 95

The Structural Basis of Corollary Discharge 97

Tight Input-Output Couplings 97

IV.   STEREOPSIS 99

Stereopsis: The Perceptual Level 99

The Cortical Neurophysiology of Stereopsis 104

Disparity-Tuned Neurons 108

Development of Visual Cortex Circuitry 113

Stereopsis: Integrating Theories 115

Theories of Hysteresis 115

V. CEREBELLAR FUNCTION 125

 The Basic Circuitry of the Cerebellar Cortex 125

  Mossy Fiber Action 128

  Braitenberg's Timing Model 130

  Marr's Learning Model 131

 Feedback and Feedforward in Cerebellar Control 133

 Cerebrocerebellar Interactions 140

 Cerebellar Projections 147

  Topography of the Spinal Projection 148

  Numerical Input-Output Relations 153

  Features of the Cerebellar Relay Systems 155

 Synergies and Cerebellar Function 157

  The Russian Perspective 157

  Boylls's Synergy Controller Model 159

Abbreviations 166

Bibliography 167

Index 199

PARTICIPANTS

Dr. Michael A. Arbib
Department of Computer and
 Information Science and Center
 for Systems Neuroscience
University of Massachusetts
Amherst, Massachusetts 01002

Dr. Colin Blakemore
Physiological Laboratory
University of Cambridge
Cambridge CB2 3EG, England

Dr. C. Curtis Boylls
Laboratory of Neurophysiology
Good Samaritan Hospital
 and Medical Center
Portland, Oregon 97210

Dr. Valentino Braitenberg
Max-Planck-Institut für
 biologische Kybernetik
Spemannstrasse 38
74 Tübingen, West Germany

Dr. Jack D. Cowan
Department of Biophysics
 and Theoretical Biology
The University of Chicago
920 East 58th Street
Chicago, Illinois 60637

Dr. Otto D. Creutzfeldt
Max-Planck-Institut für
 biophysikalische Chemie
Karl-Friedrich-Bonhoeffer Institut
D 3400 Göttingen-Nikolausberg
West Germany

Dr. Parvati Dev
Neurosciences Research Program
165 Allandale Street
Jamaica Plain, Massachusetts 02130

Dr. John C. Eccles
Laboratory of Neurobiology
State University of New York at Buffalo
4234 Ridge Lea Road
Amherst, New York 14226

Dr. Mac V. Edds, Jr.
Neurosciences Research Program
165 Allandale Street
Jamaica Plain, Massachusetts 02130

Dr. John P. Frisby
Department of Psychology
University of Sheffield
Sheffield, England

Dr. Peter H. Greene
Center for Control Research
1357 East 57th Street
Chicago, Illinois 60637

Dr. Bela Julesz
Sensory and Perceptual Processes
Bell Laboratories
600 Mountain Avenue
Murray Hill, New Jersey 07974

Dr. Bengt Larson
Institute of Physiology
University of Lund
Sölvegatan 19
S-223 62 Lund, Sweden

Dr. Donald M. MacKay
Department of Communication
University of Keele
Staffordshire ST5 5BG
Keele, England

Dr. Frank Morrell
Department of Neurology
Rush Medical College
Rush-Presbyterian-St. Luke's
 Medical Center
Chicago, Illinois 60612

Dr. Jack D. Pettigrew
Division of Biology
California Institute of Technology
Pasadena, California 91109

Dr. Enrique Ramón-Moliner
Department of Anatomy
University of Sherbrooke
 School of Medicine
Sherbrooke, Quebec, Canada

Dr. Francis O. Schmitt
Neurosciences Research Program
165 Allandale Street
Jamaica Plain, Massachusetts 02130

Dr. Cyril Stanley Smith
Department of Metallurgy and Humanities
Room 14N-317
Massachusetts Institute of Technology
Cambridge, Massachusetts 02139

Dr. John Szentágothai
1st Department of Anatomy
Semmelweis University Medical School
Tüzoltó u. 58
Budapest IX, Hungary

Dr. Hendrik Van der Loos
Institut d'Anatomie
Université de Lausanne
Faculté de Médecine
9, rue du Bugnon
CH 1011 Lausanne, Switzerland

Dr. Gerhard Werner
Department of Pharmacology
University of Pittsburgh
 School of Medicine
660 Scaife Hall
Pittsburgh, Pennsylvania 15213

Dr. Frederic G. Worden
Neurosciences Research Program
165 Allandale Street
Jamaica Plain, Massachusetts 02130

Dr. Yehoshua Y. Zeevi
Division of Engineering
 and Applied Physics
Harvard University
Pierce Hall
Cambridge, Massachusetts 02138

Note: NRP Work Session reports are reviewed and revised by participants prior to publication.

I. INTRODUCTION

This book integrates perspectives from neuroanatomy, neurophysiology, and brain theory to provide new conceptual models of neural organization. As such, it has evolved a long way from the NRP Work Session that provided the original stimulus for its writing. The Work Session had intended to explore the various uses to which the concept of hierarchy had been put in the neurosciences, with particular concern for the hierarchies that arise in those neural systems engaged in stereopsis, and those neural systems—especially the cerebellum—involved in the control of movement. At the Work Session itself, a number of workers did address the concept of hierarchy and endeavored to relate it to their work in the neurosciences; others quickly made it clear that the concept of hierarchy seemed irrelevant and not useful to the work that they were engaged in; while yet others did not mention hierarchies at all. It seemed to us that the message was clear: the concept of hierarchy was not of itself all-encompassing for the neuroscientist. However, it also seemed clear that a number of workers did find the concept important, even if other concepts proved equally significant in trying to organize the mass of data now available in brain studies, both physiological and anatomical. Thus we were determined to write a book that differs drastically in form from the actual proceedings at the Work Session. Rather than present the central discussion of hierarchies, with a large amount of apparently unrelated material, we sought to extract from the proceedings basic principles for the organization of neurons into networks and of networks into functional systems. We do not dwell on molecular or metabolic organizations of neural systems since these have been addressed in other NRP Work Sessions. Functional and structural principles are presented, respectively in Chapters II and III. Then, in Chapters IV and V we concentrate on the two areas in which we had originally hoped to find examples of hierarchical structuring: stereopsis and cerebellar function. These two chapters demonstrate that, while the concept of hierarchy by itself does not suffice to organize the material, the totality of principles presented in Chapters II and III goes a long way towards imposing order upon an almost overwhelming mass of data. They also demonstrate that there is an increasingly rich interplay between theory and experiments in the neurosciences—marked both by an increasing interest in the use of computers and mathematics by the experimentalist and an increasing willingness of the theorist to immerse himself in the intricate details of anatomy and physiology.

The principles emerged as the authors tried to combine the multiple strands of the Work Session with their own prior general observations; thus, the resultant systematization in this report had to be imposed upon the material from the Work Session rather than emerge from it. (It would be nice to take these principles and use them as a basis of a new Work Session!) In any case, we are aware that there are many details reported here that have not been assimilated into the general principles; also, there are many details to which the principles have not been accommodated. Thus, to help the reader in threading his or her way through this wealth of material, we devote the rest of this introduction to an overview of each of the four chapters that represent the body of this *Bulletin*.

A Functional Overview

In this chapter, we sought to find a number of requirements that would have to be satisfied by the controller of any system that would interact in an adaptive way with a complex environment—whether the controller be a computer inside a robot or a brain inside an animal. This led to the formulation of four general principles:

Principle 1. Theory must be action-oriented. In seeking to understand the function of any part of the brain, we must continually ask: "What interactions with its world is the animal likely to engage in?"

Principle 2. Perception is not only of "what" but also of "where." We must continually seek how the brain's activity is related to the spatial framework within which the animal interacts with its world.

Principle 3. An adaptive system must be able to correlate sensory data and actions in such a way as to update an internal model of the world. In other words, we must not only understand how neural networks can enable an animal to interact with its world, but must also understand how those networks can be structured so as to allow efficient updating with experience.

Principle 4. Organization must be hierarchical with adequate "feedback loops" to coordinate the subsystems. We present the evidence relating to the guiding principle with which the Work Session started, but note that the crude formulation—System A commands System B commands System C—cannot do justice to the variety of internal feedbacks that a system must have if high-level control is to be properly tuned to unexpected events detected at a lower level.

In addition to these four functional principles, a fifth principle is added:

Principle 5. The brain is a layered somatotopic computer. This principle lays the basis for the structural overview given in Chapter III and reminds us that these structural constraints mark a great difference between the "software" of robots that are currently being constructed and the "wetware" of an animal's brain.

In the second major section of Chapter II, the functional interaction between different regions of the brain in carrying out a sophisticated action is stressed. After a preliminary look at the somatosensory system, we emphasize Principle 2 by looking at the relationship between the perceptual computations of visual cortex and the eye-movement computations of the superior colliculus. A comparison of the somatosensory and the visual systems, with particular reference to analogies between visual and tactile search, is then made. This leads to a reassessment of the evidence on the principle of corollary discharge—how do we appropriately distinguish input that is self-generated from input that is generated by movement in the environment? The section closes with a discussion of optomotor behavior in the fly to stress the point that complex-appearing behaviors may often be explainable by relatively simple mechanisms.

In the final section of Chapter II, hierarchies of motor control are discussed in more detail. In particular, the role of feedforward and feedback in sensorimotor control is given attention, and then the minimal structural requirements and complexities of coordinated movement are determined.

A Structural Overview

If Chapter II reflects the "top-down" approach of the cybernetician, then Chapter III reflects the "bottom-up" approach of the neuroanatomist. In this chapter, principles were sought that could help us make sense of what at first appeared to be the overwhelming complexity of the neuropil.

After noting the historical importance of the idea of a neural network per se—as distinct from a syncytium—as an organizational principle before attempting to make sense of the details of neuroanatomy, we present a general discussion of the question of randomness in neural networks. Perhaps the main conclusion here is that we tend to view a network as being random to the extent that we lack a compact description of its connectivity. Thus, we may talk of randomness either because a statistical treatment of the network is sufficient for that which we wish to explain, or because the state of the art is not sufficiently developed to capture the details of that network. It would seem that the history of neuroanatomy over the past few decades has been that more and more specificity is found as we better our way of looking at the brain.

To the extent that we would discern order in the complexity of the neuropil, it seems necessary to find some intermediate unit of analysis lying between the individual neuron and the gross brain region. We seem to succeed along two different dimensions. In some structures a layer-by-layer analysis seems appropriate, with the emphasis being on the processing of two-dimensional patterns of activity as they pass from one element to another; whereas in other structures it seems most appropriate to search for modules, usually arranged to cut through a number of layers, with the emphasis here often being on lateral inhibition between different modules, although we detail other types of interaction as well.

Turning our attention away from the search for intermediate units of analysis, we engage in a comparative study of different afferent systems and find that a number of useful organizational principles seem common to the main sensory systems, although each system has specific features of its own.

Finally in our structural overview, we look at the organizational principles of internal feedback loops, seeking to distinguish these loops by the scale of interaction, going all the way from local recurrent couplings to large-scale feedback pathways.

Stereopsis

Having laid down general principles of neural organization in Chapters II and III, we tried to organize in the last two chapters the specific observations made at the Work Session on the neural mechanisms of stereopsis and on cerebellar function, especially in the control of movement. In view of the action-oriented approach stressed as Principle 1 of our functional overview, we sought in both cases to provide a general description of some overall function that was to be performed, the challenge being to see to what extent we could explain how the known neurophysiological units could be coupled to yield the given overall behavior.

Thus, in Chapter IV, we start with Julesz' experiments on the perception of random-dot stereograms to provide the framework in which we could discuss stereopsis. Then, to provide the ideas of the structural units involved, we turn to the cortical neurophysiology of stereopsis. Here our main concern is to review the data on disparity-tuned neurons, although attention is given to some of the latest ideas on the validity of the classic "center-surround cells → simple cells → complex cells → hypercomplex cells" hierarchy. There is also a review of some of the mechanisms by which the variously tuned neurons might develop during ontogeny.

Finally, a number of different models that have been developed to explain phenomena such as those reported by Julesz in the first part of this chapter are discussed. Julesz' own dipole-array model provides functional, rather than neurophysiological, mechanisms for hysteresis effects in fusion. The two-field model of Wilson and Cowan gives a more neurophysiologically plausible model of how such hysteresis effects might occur, while the Dev model of figure-ground separation builds on data on disparity-tuned neurons to suggest how inhibitory coupling might enable the various surfaces of a Julesz stereogram to "come up from the noise."

Cerebellar Function

In this final chapter, we sought to understand how the beautiful anatomy and physiology of the cerebellar cortex might help us in understanding the role that the cerebellum appears to play in modulating movement.

In the first section a quick review of the basic circuitry of the cerebellar cortex is presented; then, two models that have been based upon this circuitry are noted: the classic timing model of Braitenberg, developed on the basis of the anatomy of the cerebellar cortex before the physiological properties of the cells had been worked out, and Marr's model of possible learning in the cerebellar cortex. Ito's studies of the role of feedback and feedforward in cerebellar control also receive attention.

To place the cerebellum further in the environment of other portions of the brain, we take advantage of the elegant new ideas of Eccles on the delicate timing of the arrival of impulses in the cerebellar cortex over fast and slow pathways with the resultant coincidence of arrival of patterns in the cerebellar nuclei. We review the relationships of the vermis with the spinal cord, of the pars intermedia with both spinal cord and cerebral cortex, and of the cerebellar hemispheres with the cerebral cortex. Then, we proceed to look at the details of the projections of both mossy fibers and climbing fibers to the cerebellar cortex, noting the way in which Principle 5 of Chapter II helps us to impose structure on what had at one time been described as a uniform neural sheet.

Then, in an attempt to close the loop between overall function—the control of movement—and the details of neurophysiology and neuroanatomy, we examine some of the Russian literature on the control of movement (especially the concept of "synergy" as developed by the Moscow School) and the evidence on the intrinsic algorithms for locomotion in the spinal cord. An attempt is made to tie them together by giving the Boylls model of the cerebellum working in interaction with brainstem nuclei to modulate the playing out of the spinal algorithms.

In Retrospect

In looking back over the Work Session, and the various mutations that have been required to put together a coherent publication, we come away with the feeling that, for all its incredible complexity, the brain is slowly yielding up its secrets. If we have been disabused of any naive notions that a single organizational principle, such as that of hierarchical structuring, could provide a major key to unravelling the brain, we have, nonetheless, been encouraged by the discovery of a relatively small array of principles of neural organization—both functional and structural—that do enable us to impose order upon much available data. Perhaps even more encouragingly, they enable us to ask questions that we were unable to ask before, and these questions are so structured as to encourage the further development of cooperation between experimentalist and theorist.

II. A FUNCTIONAL OVERVIEW

General Principles for Adaptive Interaction of a Complex System with Its Environment

A common denominator throughout the discussions at the Work Session was the interaction of the organism with its environment. In this section, a number of general principles that aid us to think about the function of the brain that helps an organism to interact with its environment are provided. In Chapter IV, a process whereby an organism learns about its environment, stereopsis, i.e., the use of two eyes to see the world in depth, is discussed; in Chapter V, ideas on how the cerebellum aids the organism in acting upon its environment are presented.

Principle 1. Theory Must Be Action-Oriented

To characterize perception as the ability of a person, when shown an object, to respond by naming it is misleading. It is more appropriate to say that a person or an animal perceives its environment to the extent that it can *interact* with that environment in some reasonably structured fashion. For example, we can perceive a cat by naming it, but our perception of it often involves no conscious awareness of its being a cat per se. When it jumps on our lap while we are reading, we simply classify it by the action we take as "something to be stroked" or "something to be pushed off."

In computer jargon, where a "program" corresponds to the motor program for the generation of an action, we may say that perception of an object generally involves the gaining of access to a program rather than the execution of a program. Therefore, one perceives an object in terms of appropriate interaction with it and yet one may leave it alone. Thus, in gaining access to the program, the system, computer or animal, only gives it *potential* command. Furthermore, in the example of the cat, both the "stroke" and the "push" programs can be "accessed," but only one program can be implemented at a time. Therefore, there will be a *redundancy of potential command,* with computation required to determine which of the programs "accessed" will actually control the ensuing actions of the organism. If we have been scratched frequently by cats, the push program may take command. In his text, *The Metaphorical Brain,* Arbib (1972a, pp. 191-203) discusses various implementations of this resolution of redundancy of potential command in experimental situations where a frog snaps at only one of several flies or a vertebrate decides to fight or flee, showing how rich contacts can be made between theoretical principles and experimental data from neuro-anatomy and neurophysiology.

Principle 2. Perception Is Not Only of "What" But Also of "Where"

The primary purpose of recognizing objects is to interact with them. It is not enough to perceive the presence of a table on which to place our papers if we release our grasp of the papers some 2 meters from the table. Implicit in this viewpoint is that perception involves objects within the environment rather than the environment in toto. We have stressed that this perception may involve some simple interaction with the object rather than any detailed awareness of it. This is so, in fact, if "object" is defined in a sufficiently loose way, such as when one perceives "a row of trees" as he walks, but has no awareness of the nature or the spacing of the individual trees. Thus, our thesis must also be that most animals will perceive their world in terms of "objects," even though the nature of that perception will vary greatly from animal to animal. This theme of spatial location of object-determining surfaces rather than the location of points will play a key role in our discussion of stereopsis in Chapter IV.

Principle 3. An Adaptive System Must Be Able to Correlate Sensory Data and Actions in Such a Way as to Update an Internal Model of the World

The third principle introduces memory into our investigations. We posit that, for a complex organism (e.g., a robot or a vertebrate), experiences, skills, and memories cohere into what has been called an *internal model of the world* (Craik, 1943, 1966; MacKay, 1956, 1963; Minsky, 1961, 1965; Young, 1964; Gregory, 1969). This model is not a cardboard replica, but rather the memory structure that, for example, lets us walk into a strange room and, on the basis of visual stimuli from a brownish rhombus, know that a table is present and that we may put the papers we are carrying on that table without the risk that they will fall to the floor. In addition, *complex systems will need to modify this internal model to accommodate aspects of the environment that were not initially provided for in the model.* This could occur, for example, if such aspects have changed relatively recently. For this reason, we shall find it worthwhile to distinguish two main types of internal models. The first type encompasses relations of the organism with its immediate environment. For example, we speak of a "short-term memory" or a "short-term model." (This is a much less transient structure than the usual short-term memory described in the literature.) In the case of the reader, this might include his knowledge of the fact that he is reading the early part of this *Bulletin,* knowledge of the details of the room behind him, and awareness of his commitment to meet someone at a designated time and place in the next 24 hours. This may be contrasted with his "long-term memory" or "long-term model," which corresponds to the standing properties of his world, such as his ability to recognize an apple, ride a bicycle, or recall the details of his sixth birthday party.

Of course, it must not be thought that a new internal model is developed for every change in an object, or in its size or its position in space. Rather, the models must be flexible in a way that may be suggested by the *slide box* metaphor (Arbib, 1972a, pp. 87-121) drawn from the making of movie cartoons: Drawing each movie frame individually is too inefficient. Since a whole minute of the cartoon can run without the background being changed, one could draw the background just once. In the middle ground, there might be a tree about which nothing in particular changes during a certain period of time except its position relative to the background. It could thus be drawn on a separate slide, which could then be displaced for succeeding frames. Finally, in the foreground, it may well be that one could draw most portions of the actors for repeated use, and then position the arms, facial expressions, etc., individually for each frame. The slides can then be photographed appropriately positioned in a "slide box" for each frame, with only a few parameter changes and minimal redrawing required between each frame.

A similar strategy for obtaining an economical description of what happens over a long period of time in the brain might be used, with long-term memory corresponding to a "slide file" and short-term memory corresponding to a slide box with a selection of slides from the file. The act of perception might then be compared to the following operations on the slide box and the slide file: (1) sensory information is used to retrieve appropriate slides from the file to replace or augment those already in the slide box; (2) a comparison is made simultaneously to determine whether a newly retrieved slide fits sensory input "better" than a slide currently in the box (we shall elaborate on this suggestion in discussing Figure 3 below); (3) part of the action of the organism in changing its relationship with the environment is designed to obtain sensory input that will help update the short-term memory by deciding between "competing" slides; and (4) the sensory input helps update the long-term memory by providing data for "redrawing" and "editing" the slides. We do not imply that the above operations or processes are necessarily conscious ones.

Of course, in using the slide box metaphor one must not fall into the trap of letting terms such as "slide" impose too rigid a view of neural activity. Rather, the following should be emphasized: (1) fine perceptual acts take place against a background of brain activity; (2) small details cannot be recognized in a void; and (3) present slides strongly color the choice of each additional slide.

Unfortunately, the notion of an internal model involves higher levels of mental processes that may not be directly related to the detailed neurophysiology and anatomy discussed in the remaining chapters of this *Bulletin*. However, as Young (1964) has so elegantly argued, it does provide a framework for a long-range discussion of brain function, tying in with what some psychologists dub the "analysis-by-synthesis" view of perception. We claim that we perceive (analyze) a scene to the extent that we can synthesize a model of it. We conceptualize short-term memory not as a "tape recording" of recent input but as a synthetic representation of the whole spatiotemporal frame in which the animal moves. The process of synthesis requires extensive use of long-term memory to supply details about the environment that are not present in the immediate input. Thus, the system (human or animal) is not tied to immediate sensory cues in establishing its course of action. The system here proposed, whereby an internal model of the environment is constantly updated, enables the organism to plan ahead in resolving redundancy of potential command.

Principle 4. Organization Must Be Hierarchical with Adequate "Feedback Loops" to Coordinate the Subsystems

Hierarchical organization applies to businesses and armies as much as to brains. Just as a general is usually unaware of the details of Private Jones's movements, so must recognition of an object not be sensitive to the finest detail of light and shade. Thus, a hierarchically organized system is geared to make the most efficient use of the higher stages in the hierarchy by removing the burden of minor computation and processing to the lower stages. However, by the same token, if Private Jones succeeds in demolishing an ammunition dump, then the general must become aware of his activity. Thus, in an effective system, not only is a hierarchical arrangement valuable, but *the higher levels must constantly receive feedback about the state of implementation of their commands.*

This principle, like most of the others, must be handled with some subtlety, for the very existence of feedback can sometimes make it unclear "who is commanding whom," but the suggestion that we decompose the overall brain into subsystems will be a most important one.

Regarding the issue of the significance of built-in central patterns versus control by afferent feedback, there was general agreement at an NRP Work Session, *Central Control of Movement* (Evarts et al., 1971), that "central patterning" appears to be the basic principle of motor organization, although continuously sampled and spatially organized afferent information imparts precision and responsiveness to changing or unanticipated conditions and is probably necessary for the establishment of new specific patterns in "learned" movements.

In discussing the notions of "external feedback" versus "internal feedback" versus "corollary discharge" at that Work Session, it became apparent that the internal feedback loops, both anatomically present and physiologically active in a great many examples, could indicate that central patterning and peripheral control are not necessarily as diametrically opposed to each other as might appear. It seems, though, that it is difficult to separate conceptually the two notions of internal feedback and corollary discharge. (This topic will be discussed again below.)

The stress on such metaphors as the slide box metaphor of the internal model in discussing Principle 3 above should not hide the fact that virtually nothing is known about the anatomical connections or the physiological mechanisms involved. The participants at this Work Session appeared to agree most readily with the negative statement of Sperry (1969): "Any scheme, regardless of its complexity, in which sensory impulses are conceived to be routed through a central network system into a motor response becomes misleading." This caveat cautions us against any naive stimulus-response or unidirectional, information-flow view of neural activity. Moreover, terms such as "corticofugal control of receptors" and "internal feedback" serve to remind us that there is a continual interaction between different layers. Again, the transformations induced in each neural layer bear the marks of the animal's history, both as an individual and as a member of the species. Whether we talk of learning or evolution, we seek to understand the underlying processes of adaptation that have led to an organism's ability to interact with its environment.

Advantages and Disadvantages

It is worth noting some advantages and disadvantages of a hierarchical type of command system arranged to make the most efficient use of the highest levels of command by reducing the complexity of their computations. Some of the advantages include the following: (1) more time is available for creative problem solving (planning) to deal with novel situations; (2) more space is available in that more "memories" can be stored if their description does not deal with all the little details; and (3) new tasks (or similar tasks) are more easily and rapidly learned as long as they are not too difficult. Having local control also allows specific, uncomplicated actions (like withdrawing a hand from a hot stove) to be performed very quickly. Another advantage is that the information flow is substantially reduced in comparison to that of an organization that has only one level of command. Some of the disadvantages are as follows: if our interest is only in the efficiency of the motor part of movement (i.e., ignoring central, computational complexity), we should be able to find a better pattern and sequence of muscle activation if our computation included every detail of the situation. Just as rubbing the stomach while patting the head is hard, so the behavior possible to the animal is drastically reduced in degrees of freedom by the hierarchical arrangement. Thus, some peculiar environmental change might result in situations that the animal cannot meet. Also, learning unusual tasks may be hard (e.g., learning to walk differently as in modern dance). Nonetheless, it is clear, both for an animal and a robot, that most tasks will lend themselves to decomposition into familiar subtasks, and that level-by-level refinement of tasks will normally be vastly more efficient than any attempt to replace a high-level command with a sequence of machine language instructions.

Hierarchy of Levels of Description

In addition to the hierarchical organizations embodied in Principle 4, there is a hierarchy of levels of description. Four such levels of increasing details are: (1) overall functional behavior, (2) decomposition of functional behavior in terms of gross anatomy versus decomposition in terms of subfunctions (unfortunately, since the results of these two decompositions may differ, we must then suggest how groups of subfunctions are related to (i.e., played out across) groups of substructures), (3) layer-by-layer analysis of nuclei and cortical regions, and (4) details of local neural circuitry and function.

The study of stereopsis (Chapter IV) starts with a clear functional description (i.e., Level 1) of locating objects in space and then jumps to the details of neural activity in visual cortex (Level 4). Here, the task is to find a theory, essentially at Level 3, that may guide our analysis of neural connections at Level 4 by suggesting how neurons of known behavior may cooperate to yield stereopsis. On the other hand, the discussion of the role of the cerebellum in the control of movement (Chapter V) begins with an anatomical decomposition of the cerebellum into its cortical regions and its nuclei (Level 2) without our having, at present, a clear notion of the overall cerebellar function (Level 1)—a deficit that an analysis of the Russian work on the control of movement (see below) may begin to remedy. Since we have a very good view of Level 4, experiments at Level 1 are needed to give overall behavioral descriptions and a theory that can then knit the manifold details of cellular anatomy and physiology into a meaningful control system. A final understanding of the cerebellum will probably involve answering questions such as: "How do you 'choose' a movement?" "How do you 'decide' how to carry it out?" "What 'subroutines' may be called upon in the spinal cord?" It will also require a deep analysis of the evolutionary interdependence of motor and sensory nuclei.

Hierarchy of Anatomical Structures

Regarding the usage of Principle 4, a few words are in order about hierarchies of levels of control. For example, a popular notion is a hierarchy of anatomical structures with three main levels: (1) a cortex providing strategies and, perhaps, long-term memory, (2) a midbrain or brainstem assembling the strategies, and (3) a spinal cord and brainstem executing built-in routines. But functions need not be anatomically segmented so rigidly. For example, the motor cortex is, in a sense, more "automatic" than some brainstem regions. Again, there may be hierarchical levels in an evolutionary sense, and yet the function is distributed at all levels. For example, the function of the superior colliculus is modified by thalamic and cortical structures so that their mutual interaction provides more sophisticated visuomotor activity (see the section on "Multiple Representations"). Two levels, A and B (such as cortex and superior colliculus), may be so intimately interlinked that one cannot even make statements such as "Level A commands Level B while Level B informs Level A," since it might be equally valid to say "Level B commands Level A and Level A informs Level B." For this reason, McCulloch's (1945) term *heterarchy** has become popular among some workers in artificial intelligence (see, e.g., Minsky and Papert, 1972).

Similarly, in going from sensory to motor areas, a hierarchy of anatomical structures appears to exist. One observes a continuum of increasingly abstract representation of sensory information. However, this can also be interpreted as an increased specification of motor programs, thus raising doubts about the ordering of these structures in a hierarchy. Note that, while there seems to exist more symmetry in horizontal intracortical connections, there is asymmetry perpendicular to the cortex. A naive structural view would thus suggest a mainly vertical organization, and yet we have a transcortical model of information flow. To understand anatomy, we must understand function—physics does not tell us what a beer can opener does!

Principle 5. The Brain Is a Layered Somatotopic Computer

Unfortunately, too many neuroscientists are still thinking in terms of single-electrode results and what may be happening at any given point; few appear to be concerned about two- and three-dimensional patterns of neural activity, and with what meaningful information may be conveyed by such patterns (cf. Creutzfeldt et al., 1971).

The relationship between two layers of cells connected by fibers, such as the body surface receptors and sensorimotor cortex, is called somatotopic (from the Greek *soma* for body and *topos* for place)

---

*Heterarchy is defined in the dictionary as "rule by aliens," but McCulloch uses the term in the sense of "distributed rule" as opposed to the "rule from a single apex" of hierarchical structures, such as the head of a church body.

when it preserves approximate information about place on the body as we move from receptors to the central nervous system, with the representation biased by the amount of information that each receptor region can contribute to the animal's activity. (Compare the discussion of the work of Van der Loos below and Figure 18). Apparent discontinuities in the "homuncular" shapes of most representation maps of body periphery in the centers (cerebral cortex, cerebellar cortex, thalamus, etc.) can be understood and interpreted as topological transformations (see Werner, 1970). It is important to realize that most other connections between nerve centers are subject to similar rules of topographical order, although they no longer have direct relations to body periphery. Such topographical orderliness is, nevertheless, also referred to as *somatotopic* with good reason, since erosion (see the section on "Multiple Representations") of the topographic map in the centers not directly connected with the periphery does not abolish order of connection but leads only to more complex maps in which body space, originally represented, loses its primary importance. The term "somatotopically organized" is used to remind us that, even though position on the body does not provide the key coordinate for interpreting activity in layers of the brain far from the periphery, nonetheless, this type of map or positional code will help us to understand what is going on in these layers.

The straightforward (isomorphic) representation of body periphery in primary sensory and motor centers corresponds to reality only on a gross scale. Whenever we are looking for the finer details, we come to recognize that the same spot of the periphery is represented centrally in many different ways and in different contexts, often over very different routes and relay mechanisms, within the same gross map. An impressive example of this will be given in the projection of the forelimb to the anterior lobe of the cerebellum in Chapter V. A structural analysis of Principles 4 and 5 (hierarchy and somatotopy) will be given in the section on "Layer-by-Layer Analysis" in Chapter III.

Neuroscientists have repeatedly speculated about the causes of, and the developmental mechanisms bringing about, the somatotopic relations. The most general and overriding expression of somatotopy is the crossing of neural pathways, present in many invertebrates (generally on a minute scale), that phylogenetically has become the major architectural principle of the vertebrate CNS. Most classical authors, particularly Ramón y Cajal (1909, 1911), have approached this problem from the somewhat ambiguous aspect of teleology. Even recently, when the crossing of the pathways became an issue of paramount importance from split brain experiments (Gazzaniga, 1970; Milner, 1974; Sperry, 1974), understanding of the real significance of this basic architectural principle remained obscure. An investigation into the development of the frequently observed crossed projections between the periphery and the lowest centers (labeled elementary crossings) led Szentágothai and Székely (1956b) to assume that the reverse projections, with a crossing in the middle, were based on what they called the "camera lucida" or "pinhole camera" principle of neural connections. It was their contention that neuroblasts have a primary axis orientation determining the direction in which the axon starts to grow. Although further orientation of axonal growth is subject to a great many different secondary factors modifying the direction of growth, as has been admirably analyzed by Weiss (1950b), the primary axis orientation of the axons largely determines the basic geometrical pattern of the projection. Axons tend to grow in a straight direction, as long as they are not induced by other forces to deviate; hence, the similarity between neural and optical projections justifies use of the metaphorical expression "camera lucida." The crossings of the neural pathways over the midline were, in the final analysis, found to follow the same basic principle, and it was pointed out by Szentágothai and Székely (1956b) that, in a developing and growing tissue mass of complex shape and bilateral symmetry, crossings of many pathways are unavoidable, and the mentioned causal factors operating in the elementary kinds of projections would also be at the very roots of somatotopies in general.

On the other hand, an elegant evolutionary explanation by Braitenberg (1965a) is more in the spirit of this section. He suggests that, if we regard smell as the dominant sense of a hypothetical protovertebrate, then the uncrossed olfactory input coupled to a crossed motor map makes sense: for example, food smelled on the right side will cause an increased motor activity on the left side, causing the animal to turn in the direction of the food. Young (1964) has hypothesized that internal maps must be in register. Braitenberg argues that the motor map is far more detailed than the olfactory input, so later evolving sensory systems should be mapped in registry with the motor rather than the olfactory map.

Multiple Representations

What is the significance of multiple representations of the sensory inputs that occur in the various visual cortical areas? Can hierarchies provide a rationale for multiple representation? What do we mean when we talk of "feedback in a hierarchy"? To focus on these questions, a more detailed look at the problem of internal "modeling" of the extracorporeal world is needed.

The visual cortex of mammals operates on a global feature space, whereas in the frog tectum there is local feature domination. We can, to a crude first approximation, talk about two visual systems: the "where" system in the midbrain and the "what" system in the visual cortex. Thus, the spinal cord is controlled by the midbrain and the midbrain by the cortex. But it is also possible to have heterarchical organization in the sense of lower level systems taking command, which brings us to the question of the role of eye movement in vision. The superior colliculus controls the movement of the eyes, but one can also have eye movements controlled by hypotheses generated internally. Here, eye movements subserve the process of comparing what we see with an internally generated model. For example, when asked to memorize chessboards, the eye movements of nonchess players are random, whereas eye movements of chess players are characterized by "strategy-linked," scan-path patterns (Tikhomirov and Poznyanskaya, 1966-1967).

The evolution of a "stimulus" during processing may be considered as an evolution from "pointillism" to "representation"—a transformation (not without internal feedbacks) from the neural activity corresponding to stimuli impinging on a receptor surface to that corresponding to action-oriented cognitive strategies such as chessboard comprehension. To prevent our exposition from being too modality-bound, we start by comparing somatosensory representation with visual representation, noting the dissimilarities and boundary conditions. Whether in looking at a picture or tactually exploring a shape, the system must explore the nonfamiliar object with a *series* of *parallel* processings.

The Somatosensory System

Object manipulation plays a major role in the acquisition of stimulus information for tactile apprehension of object quality and

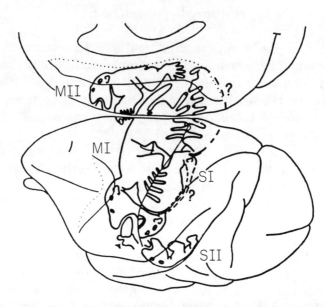

Figure 1. Diagram of monkey cortex showing locations and general plans of organization of the supplementary motor (MII), the precentral motor (MI), the postcentral tactile (SI), and the second sensory (SII) areas. The latter (SII) lies largely on the upper bank of the Sylvian fissure adjacent to the insula and the auditory area on the lower bank (not illustrated). [Modified from Woolsey, 1958]

shape (Gibson, 1962). In "active touch," the observer seems to be trying to obtain mechanical events on the skin in various combinations and places, thereby generating a series of "snapshots," each of which consists of a particular finger posture and a set of object-skin contact points. This sequence of snapshots results from conjoint, though distinctly identifiable, activities: shaping the hand while held stationary to grasp the object and displacing the hand along contours and surfaces. The currently available evidence from primate behavioral studies suggests that this "active touch" is dependent on the integrity of the somatosensory cortex.

   Woolsey and his colleagues (1942; Woolsey and Fairman, 1946) identified two somatosensory cortical projection areas (SI and SII) and argued from circumstantial evidence (notably the proximity to phylogenetically old brain structures) that SII was a more primitive cortical area (see Figure 1). Sanides (1970) arrived at a similar conclusion from cytoarchitectonic and evolutionary considerations. SII neurons receive purely cutaneous afferent input from bilateral receptive fields (Whitsel et al., 1969). For the latter reason, their activity remains ambiguous with regard to the lateralization of a stimulus on the body surface. In

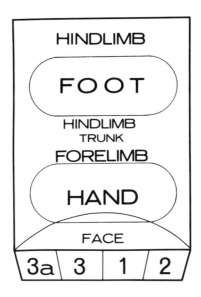

Figure 2. Schematic display of the body topography in SI of the macaque in reference to the cytoarchitectonic areas 3a, 3, 1, and 2. [Modified from Dreyer et al., 1974]

SI, which is composed of the cytoarchitectonic areas 3a, 3, 1, and 2, an orderly map of the body is obtained, as shown schematically in Figure 2 (see Werner, 1972).

The different submodalities of somesthesis distribute differentially in this cortical map, in accord with cytoarchitectural areas: area 3a receives afferent input from muscle receptors; areas 3 and 1 receive cutaneous input; and area 2 receives input from joint afferents and slowly adapting cutaneous receptors. At least for the hindlimb projection, there is also evidence that different regions in the cortical map are supplied by different afferent tracts: fasciculus gracilis of the dorsal columns contributes primarily to the representation of the distal portion of the limb, while afferents from the proximal portions of the limb reach their cortical destination primarily via the dorsolateral funiculus of the spinal cord (Dreyer et al., 1974).

In spite of this multiplicity of submodalities and spinal pathways, there is one common principle that underlies the mapping process: groups of primary afferents are arranged within each dermatome in such a manner that the peripheral receptive fields of each group of afferents form characteristic sequences on the body. As far as the mapping process is concerned, these "dermatomal trajectories" constitute subassemblies of afferents, each remaining preserved as the elementary unit of which the map in SI is composed (Werner and

Whitsel, 1968). As a consequence of this essentially topological mapping process, metric relations between regions on the body are not preserved, and the same body regions may project to different places in the cortical map, each time in different local contexts and with different local neighborhood relations.

The significance of SI for active touch can be attributed to two circumstances: in the first place, SI contains neurons that signal the direction of stimulus motion on the skin and are, therefore, capable of supplying information about the movement of object contours that are in contact with the skin (Whitsel et al., 1972); secondly, SI has extensive reciprocal connections with the motor cortex (area 4). Both factors may be assumed to be of importance for initiation and guidance of the grasping and displacing movements that constitute active touch.

The first step in the outward projection from SI along its intracortical sensory path is directed to the adjacent area 5 in the parietal lobe. It is characterized by two significant changes: The topographic parcellation in SI is partially discarded, thus initiating the bringing together of somesthetic information from parts of the body that were distinctly kept apart in the SI map (Jones and Powell, 1970). Moreover, submodalities begin to converge and single neurons in area 5 can now signal particular combinations of joint positions and skin impressions (Duffy and Burchfiel, 1971). It is as if the discrete sense data acquired by the combined operation of SI and motor cortex were regrouped in area 5 and, thereby, converted into a data structure that is more conducive to the formation of an internal representation of the stimulus space than was the discrete projection of body regions and modalities in SI.

Comparison of Different Sensory Systems

According to Werner, the following comparison between the cortical connections of primary sensory areas for vision and touch may point to significant functional differences: somatic sensory and visual areas, each, project in a first step to a local region, i.e., the somatic cortex projects to area 5 in the parietal lobe, and area 17 projects to circumstriate cortex of the occipital lobe; these primary sensory areas also project to a portion of premotor cortex in the frontal lobes. But the primary visual area remains isolated from the rest of the cortex in not receiving any fibers returning from elsewhere, whereas there are heavy reciprocal connections between somatic areas and motor cortex (area 4) (Jones and Powell, 1970). Moreover, the motor cortex receives input from the visual system indirectly from the areas beyond the striate cortex (cf. Weiskrantz, 1972).

This difference in connection patterns seems to correspond to distinct differences in the information processing capabilities of somatic and visual cortex, although both sensory systems are concerned with the acquisition of information on objects in extracorporeal space. For example, in vision, depth information can be obtained by stereopsis without the need for movement; on the other hand, in the somato-sensory system, movement is essential for localization and definition of object contours, thus indicating a high degree of interdependence of somatosensory and motor activity. This may also account for the fact that activity of neurons in the somatic cortex is apparently much more subject to variation depending on the behavioral context than seems to be the case with neurons in the striate cortex (cf. Werner, 1974).

Similarly, it may be appropriate to compare the role of the glabrous skin of the hand as the organ of palpation with the fovea for the extraction of stimulus detail: the surrounding skin in the one case and the visual periphery in the other guide the fingers and the fovea to attention-worthy regions.

On moving away from the primary sensory area (backwards into area 5), an erosion of the strict topography in cortical representation of body space takes place. Convergence from several joints is a prominent feature of area 5 (Duffy and Burchfiel, 1971), and "stimulus space" rather than "body space" appears to be represented. Werner stressed the similarity, in this respect, between the primary somatosensory cortex (areas 3, 1, and 2) and area 17, which is retinotopically arranged: the projection eventually undergoes in both sensory systems a similar erosion of topography at secondary or more remote regions of representation while at the same time more complex and specialized features are extracted. In the cat, area 17 is almost certainly involved in stereopsis. In the monkey, area 18 specializes in stereopsis (though what Hubel and Wiesel (1970) called area 18 is probably anterior to true area 18). The superior temporal sulcus is involved in movement detection without regard to shape (Dubner and Zeki, 1971); area 5 signals conjunctive stimuli, e.g., touch *and* position. Strangely, there does not appear to exist a simple topographic map in the auditory cortex (Evans, 1968). However, it appears as if auditory space as such was mapped, suggesting that the spatial organization is, indeed, analogous in all main sensory systems (see, for instance, the work of Morrell (1972) on the neural representation of acoustical space).

In fair agreement with the observations in primary visual cortex by Hubel and Wiesel (1968) and in primary auditory cortices by Evans (1968), little information processing appears to occur in lamina IV of SI, which receives the specific sensory afferents, other than some rather specific convergence of the probably exclusively excitatory afferents. (The possibilities of an inhibitory "shaping" of the arriving afferent pattern will be discussed later in Chapter III.) But response properties of the neurons in SI become more complex in more superficial or deeper layers of the sensory cortices. An analogy between the visual (Pettigrew et al., 1968b) and the somatosensory (Whitsel et al., 1972) cortex is also fair with respect to the highest incidence of fast spontaneous activity in the cells of lamina IV, while becoming lower with increasing specificity of trigger features in laminas III and V.

A general principle of cortical representation that might be deduced from Werner's studies on movement detectors of the skin is the possibility of monitoring motor behavior for the exploration of object contours. This would be analogous to the alleged role of visual feature detectors in eye movement control (Blakemore, 1970b). The anatomical substrate of the guidance of motor behavior for the acquisition of tactile information by movement detectors could be ensured by the reciprocal connections between the somatosensory and somatomotor areas referred to earlier in this section.

As a related system, consider Van der Loos's study of cortical barrels of the vibrissae system of the mouse. The vibrissae are sensitive detectors of movement and may provide the substrate for sensory guidance of motor exploratory behavior. (This will be discussed in detail in the section on "Large-Scale Organoid Modules" in Chapter III.) Similar barrel structures are found in the raccoon whose cortex actually has little bumps corresponding to the eminences in the palm and to the finger pads. Humans do not show such a barrel structure for fingers.

In the lateral line system, the hair cell receptors detect some aspect, mechanical or electrical, of the immediate environment. Every other hair cell detects movement in one direction and the alternate hair cells detect movement in the opposite direction.

The important points in the above discussion can be summarized as follows: (1) The initial mapping of sensory information corresponds to the body surface or the retina surface. This neighborhood preservation (i.e., two points that are close on the retina are also close in the visual cortex) is important for any simple computation of how to move so as to obtain more information about the input, i.e., "foveation." (2) Within a neighborhood, the same input is repeatedly available, each time in a different context. The context may differ as to modality, features, etc., which permits computation of a number of features and relations. (3) Further analysis must involve loss of information about actual localization of input but must extract coincidence or conjunction between different stimuli as we go from a sensory representation to a motor representation.

Eye Movements and Visual Perception

As expressed above under "General Principles for Adaptive Interaction of a Complex System with Its Environment," the perceptual system is viewed as a hierarchically organized system that uses short-term memory (a current "model of the world") constructed from current input information and associations from long-term memory. A point of importance here is that not only effector subsystems (that generate movements) but also preprocessing subsystems (arrays of feature detectors) are seen as being controllable by the perceptual system. Thus, we hypothesize that the "features" being utilized by the system change according to the perceptual task that is being carried out.

To substantiate the role of sensory exploration in perception, consider a plausible scheme for the control of eye movements during visual perception (Figure 3; Didday and Arbib, 1973). As is well known, the afferent signals from the eye (A) traverse (among many others) two distinct pathways: the geniculostriate pathway leading to

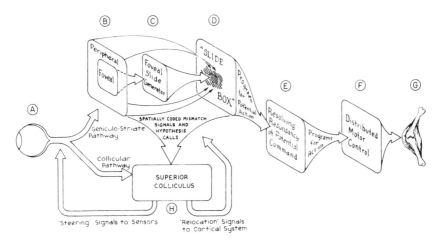

Figure 3. A scheme for cerebral-collicular interaction in the control of eye movements during visual perception. [Didday and Arbib, 1973]

the visual cortex (caricatured by region B) and the collicular pathway leading to the superior colliculus (H). Recognizing that this dichotomy of destinations is not so strict in real visual systems and that there are more than two destinations for visual projections, Arbib and Didday (1971), nevertheless, feel that it is premature to incorporate these details if one is to achieve a testable model.

The cortical visual information is processed to yield what Arbib and Didday (1971) have termed "output feature clusters" (OFC's). These are internal encodings of high-level *motor* commands that, if released, act in concert to produce an appropriate response. Didday and Arbib (1973) hypothesize that there is a region (D, called the slide box for reasons elaborated above) that holds the updated encoding of the "percepts" of a scene as a spatially coded array of output feature clusters. (Where D is actually embodied in the cortex is still open to question. Recognizing the functions necessary to the model, Didday and Arbib still leave open a number of anatomical correlations.) Box E, then, "resolves the redundancy of potential command" in the array of OFC's, activating the distributed motor control (F) to recode the activated program in terms of the motoneuron activity that will control the skeletal musculature (G). Henceforth, ignore the output system (E, F, and G) uninvolved in the control of eye movements and, instead, concentrate on the interaction between the cortical visual system (B, C, and D) and the midbrain visual system (H) in perception. One must also consider transformations that occur in E, F, and G to keep the internal model in register with the action frame of the organism.

The premise that evolution (in the guise of comparative studies) can provide essential clues in our study of the human brain suggests that the human visual system be modeled as a two-level system, in which the superior colliculus plays a role akin to that played by the tectum in the frog (namely, orienting the system to local features of the environment), in addition to a new role played in interaction with the cortical mechanisms (B, C, and D) that construct the organism's model of its current environment.

The slide box (D) is to be thought of as containing an overall pattern of activation built up by the "insertion" of OFC's corresponding to different objects or well-defined subscenes in the environment. This insertion is posited to be the task of the "foveal slide generator" (C). Here, the crucial observation is that human vision is acute foveally but relatively diffuse peripherally, suggesting that elicitation from long-term memory of all but the most familiar OFC's would require cuing by matching an array of foveal features. Clearly, then, the visual system must be able to "steer" the eye to bring such cuing arrays of features into the fovea so that system C may retrieve the OFC's for insertion into the slide box (D).

Think of the slides as being two-sided, with the input side appropriate for matching with sensory features, while the output side is so configured that it provides appropriate motor program signals to E and F. At any time, the slide box will be partially filled, corresponding to the cumulative effect of past insertions. Of this activity, only a fraction needs to correspond to current visual input; this is indicated in Figure 3 by the regions with horizontal hatching (foveal input) and diagonal hatching (peripheral input) in D. The activity on the input side of each slide is compared with the current visual input from the external world to see how well they correspond. Didday and Arbib consider, as part of the specification of an OFC, the details of some areas to be crucial, and those of other areas to be unimportant. (If the OFC currently active in the slide box is, indeed, the correct one, this does not rule out that the foveal slide generator may seize upon these details to elicit another OFC.) Thus, a mismatch of OFC and visual input in a given region of the spatial frame increases with discrepancy between the visual input and the input side of the OFC, but decreases to the extent that that region is given low weight in the slide specification. As a result of this comparison process, a spatial array of mismatch signals is "played down" from the cortex upon the superior colliculus, in spatial register with the "local feature" map transmitted by the collicular pathway. A third map played down in spatial register upon the colliculus may be called the "hypothesis-confirmation" map. The visual cues reaching foveal slide generator (C) may be able to elicit several different slides or hypotheses, but further information is required to confirm or disconfirm these several hypotheses. Often, the approximate spatial location of decisive information can be determined from the current activity in C, and it is then posited that it is signals of this kind, weighted as to the strength they would have in confirming or disconfirming a hypothesis, that make up the hypothesis-confirmation map that provides the third spatial input array to the superior colliculus in the model. There will also be contributions to this map from the slide box—our current knowledge of the environment may suggest the presence of other objects in the environment even in the absence of visual stimuli cuing the object at that time.

Before suggesting how the three spatial arrays are combined in the superior colliculus, brief mention of two other mechanisms required for the proper functioning of the cortical system (B, C, and D) should be made. First, proper control of the pathways between B, C, and D is required to "relocate" appropriately the signals to the cortical system, despite varying orientations of the eyes (cf. the discussion of the "reafference principle" of von Holst and Mittelstaedt under "Corollary Discharge"), while noting (as in the papers of MacKay referred to below) that one cannot expect such reafference to yield more than approximate compensation. Didday and Arbib (1973) suggest that it is the decomposition of slide box activity in terms of OFC's corresponding to objects that then allows the necessary fine tuning, since an OFC can then be transformed (or be transformed with respect to) in toto until sufficient register is obtained, given an initial rough transformation. (The "co-moving sets" that Arbib (1969) introduced to allow translation in toto of arrays of activation representing subautomata within a tessellation may well provide an appropriate first approximation to a formalism for describing the transformation of slides.)

Occasionally, of course, an object will appear so unexpectedly different from a new perspective that a new slide must be found to represent it. Thus, the model specifies the following: (1) the foveal slide generator (C) may generate several OFC's before actually inserting one in the slide box; and (2) another resolution of redundancy of potential command mechanism must be provided to evaluate the slides suggested by C in comparison to the foveal visual input, the current slide in the horizontally hatched region of D, and the overall context established by the current totality of activation in the slide box.

To complete the model-schema, only the function of the superior colliculus (H) needs to be specified. In Didday's (1970) model of the frog tectum (see also Arbib, 1972a, pp. 197-200), the tectal input was caricatured as a spatial array coding "foodness." It was posited that a layer of computation resolved redundancy of potential command within this array, and that the resolved output played upon a distributed motor control to cause the frog to orient towards and snap at the fly whose "foodness" achieved actual "command" of the system. In the current model, Didday and Arbib (1973) posit that the superior colliculus has a computing layer that resolves redundancy of potential command in its input array in precisely the manner in which Didday's model of the tectum resolves redundancy, but that the resolved output plays upon a distributed motor control to cause a saccade of the eyes towards the region of the visual field in spatial register with the region of the input array that achieved actual command of the system. It only remains to specify the nature of the input array to the redundancy of potential command resolver.

In each region of the collicular input array, there are three types of signals: a "low-level feature" signal from the collicular pathway and "mismatch" and "hypothesis-confirmation" signals from the cortical system. These are combined to yield one "attention-worth" signal. The exact formula for the combination need not concern us here; the crucial point is that it is monotonic in all three variables, and that the relative importance of these three variables can be changed, depending on what we shall loosely refer to as the "affective state" of the organism. For example, when we are "jittery," the collicular pathway may dominate, i.e., "we are easily distracted," but, when we are "daydreaming," the hypothesis-confirmation signal may dominate visual perception to the virtual exclusion of mismatch and collicular pathway signals.

The overall import of this model is that different regions of, and beyond, the visual field will compete for the attention of the organism. The evaluation of the attention worth of the region will depend upon the intrinsic novelty (such as an unexpected flash of light) of the low-level features of the region, the degree of mismatch between high-level features of the region and the current internal model of that region, and the extent to which the organism posits that the region contains perceptually important information. Moreover, collicular input will be depressed in regions for which the slide box contains OFC's that have received a high degree of confirmation. The regions then compete in a structure akin to that provided by Didday (1970) in his model of the tectum. If, and when, a region emerges as the "winner" from such a resolution of redundancy of potential command, the superior colliculus will both direct a saccade of the eyes towards this region and send a "relocation" signal to the cortical system to ensure that foveal input will be routed towards the appropriate region of the slide box.

Corollary Discharge

The general problem of the so-called corollary discharge, which is obviously intimately linked with internal feedback loops, was also discussed in much detail at the NRP Work Session on *Central Control of Movement* (Evarts et al., 1971). However, even the careful confrontation (at that Work Session) of the classical views of Helmholtz (1867), Sperry (1950), von Holst and Mittelstaedt (1950), and of the more recent views of MacKay (1965) and Teuber (1967), with the pertinent data from contemporary neurophysiology does not provide any satisfactory structural-functional explanation. It appears, in fact, that there is no universal principle valid for various levels of neural function. The discussion of the previous section clearly shows that there are situations in which a one-dimensional subtraction is too simple, whereas the work of Szentágothai and Székely (1956a) suggests that certain experiments on salamanders can be explained without invoking corollary discharge at all. Briefly, Szentágothai and Székely (1956a) noted that the fundamental observations by Sperry (1950) on the circling motion of eye-reversed fish and by von Holst and Mittelstaedt (1950) on the spinning of head-rotated flies, on which the concept of corollary discharge partially rests, are essentially a "pseudo-problem." On analyzing the optokinetic behavior of "one eye"- or "double eye"-reversed newts and their assumed inverse visual projections in detail (including some speculations on the possible underlying neuronal mechanisms), Szentágothai and Székely (1956a) concluded that the observations are exactly what would be expected on the basis of the most rigid, classical reflex principles. Hence, there would be no reason to assume any new principle of neural organization. Furthermore, the alleged inability of amphibia to adapt to the reversed sensory projections resulting from eye reversal was shown to be incorrect, all observations being explicable on the basis of assuming two exactly matching errors: erroneous (reverse) localization of the prey and reverse visual feedback during the assault. Whenever the exact matching of the two errors is broken, either by having a nonreversed portion of the visual field (which is, of course, not used in the behavioral test situations for the localization of the prey) or by the possibility of moving the eyes separately (i.e., the position of the eye to the head is not fixed as in most cases of experimentally induced visual field reversal), the animal quickly becomes aware of the reversal of the visual field. Since there is no cessation of attempts at attacking if the visual field reversal is complete and the position of the eye relative to the head is fixed, the explanation has to be that (1) the "matching of errors" and (2) the generation of corrective movements (based on external feedback) are a built-in part of the lower reflex mechanism.

As made clear above, Arbib and Szentágothai do not deny the significance of the concept of the corollary discharge. However, they suggest that it might be applicable only to voluntary or spontaneous movements, a possibility already hinted at in the *NRP Bulletin* by

Evarts and his colleagues (1971, p. 111). If the lower, partly reflex mechanisms with their known simpler feedback loops are incorporated into the concept of corollary discharge, one could easily be trapped into making simplistic "pseudoneuronal" hypotheses about this fundamental phenomenon. Most misconceptions arise from trying to combine speculations on external feedbacks of the lower mechanisms, i.e., the basic phenomena observed by Sperry (1950) and by von Holst and Mittelstaedt (1950), with the environmental stability observed during voluntary eye movement. The latter phenomenon points, indeed, towards some fundamental neural mechanisms that, probably for the time being, are best explained by MacKay's hypothesis that information from the motor centers is used by the CNS to evaluate the evidence afforded by sensory reafference from exploratory movements. For a reconciliation of his view with those of von Holst and Mittelstaedt, see MacKay and Mittelstaedt (1974). In fact, on the cortical level (areas 17 and 18), no signs of a corollary discharge due to the eye movement itself were discovered with single-neuron recordings (Creutzfeldt et al., 1972). These authors found, however, that the fast movement of an image across the retina during a saccade inhibits transmission through the retinal, the geniculate, and the cortical networks so that an orderly neuronal representation of the retinal image is wiped out during the saccade.

Optomotor Behavior in the Fly

Braitenberg gave an illuminating example of optomotor behavior based on work from the Max Planck Institute for Biological Cybernetics at Tubingen (Gotz, 1968; Reichardt, 1973), which illustrates how apparently complex behavior may occasionally be reduced to a set of surprisingly simple mechanisms. Consider the navigation of a fly in a room. A naive description of its behavior in simple terms would be as follows: the fly will sometimes fly a straight course or a tortuous path, apparently dictated by its whims or, if you wish, by the rules of its exploratory behavior. Then, it seems to isolate an object from the background, for it directs its attention to the lamp suspended from the ceiling. It decides to land there and definitely turns its course to that object. Just before it lands there, another set of actions begins: the landing gear is put out (the legs are stretched forward) and the flying speed is reduced. Finally, the fly comes to rest on the surface of the lampshade. Much of this complex behavior may be a simple

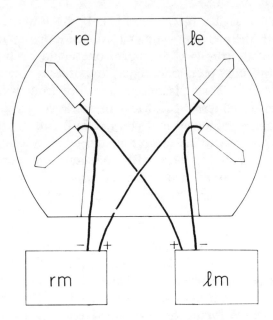

Figure 4. Diagrammatic front view of a fly. The arrows in the eye represent sets of motion detectors of two different orientations. The output of the motion detectors is fed directly into the motor system with a plus (flight muscles are activated) or minus (flight muscles are inhibited) sign. re = right eye; le = left eye; rm = right flight muscle; lm = left flight muscle. [Braitenberg]

consequence of the fly's optomotor reactions, in other words, of its perception of movement in the visual field and of a simple pattern of connections between the movement detectors and the flight muscles.

Each of the motion detectors, which are distributed over the entire visual field, is activated by input from two neighboring channels of the compound eye. They are directional and are oriented in at least two different directions. In fact, some effects on the flight navigation of the fly are maximal for horizontal movement in the visual field and absent for vertical movement, while for some other effects the converse is true. This is not compatible with movement detectors of one orientation only. Let us suppose that they are oriented in the direction of the arrows of Figure 4, obliquely upwards and backwards and obliquely downwards and backwards in each eye (in reality the situation is certainly more complex since at least another arrow with opposite orientation would have to be added to each arrow in the same eye). Each of the arrows stands for a large set of movement detectors, perhaps one for each ommatidium (for each of the 3000 channels of the compound eye). Now let the output of each set of movement

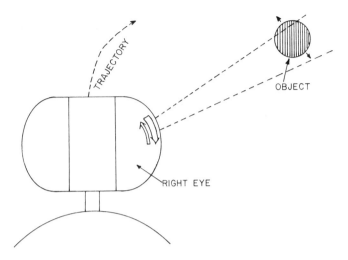

Figure 5. Top view of a fly orienting towards an isolated object. The object, which is wiggling back and forth, elicits optomotor reactions of opposite direction and different magnitude (symbolized by the large and small arrows in the right eye). The net effect is a curved trajectory that makes the animal turn towards the object. [Braitenberg]

detectors be connected with the apparatus regulating wing beat amplitude during flight (supposing that nothing else changes in the wing beat) according to the scheme of Figure 4. The fibers from the movement detectors activate or inhibit the flight muscles as indicated by the plus and minus signs and the following is observed: (1) Horizontal movement to one side will be seen by both movement-detector sets of one eye, but not by those of the other eye. The effect on the muscular system will be such as to make the flight asymmetric: the animal will turn towards the same side. (2) Vertical movement upwards will increase the strength of the two "motors" bilaterally and movement downwards will depress them symmetrically.

These effects can actually be observed in optomotor behavior and can be understood as a mechanism for the optical stabilization of flight. (There is more to it; the foreground-background reference ("Vordergrund-Hintergrund-Beziehung") of the Gestalt psychologists may also be reduced to optomotor reactions.) Consider in Figure 5 another aspect of the movement-detecting mechanism. Again, the two arrows represent movement detectors, but the one representing movement from front to back (the big arrow) is more powerful than the one in the opposite direction (the small arrow). Suppose that each arrow will elicit a turning movement of the animal in the corresponding direction. An object wiggling back and forth in the visual field of the fly will therefore elicit alternate optomotor reactions in the opposite directions, with one prevailing over the other so that the net effect will be a turn towards that object. Instead of the wiggling of the object, a wiggling of the head will have the same effect. If the difference between the two opposite optomotor reactions is itself variable as a function of the position of the input in the visual field, a complicated field of forces will arise that will make flies orient towards objects in their visual field, and the tortuous trajectories can be nicely explained. Finally, it is not difficult to imagine a pattern of connections between the movement detectors and the muscles of the legs that make the fly "extend the landing gear" for a rapid radially divergent movement in the front part of the visual field, such as the fly perceives when it approaches a landing surface. In a somewhat optimistic view, then, the entire trajectory of the fly, which we have previously observed and naively interpreted, can be predicted from its initial velocity and direction, when we know the structure of its visual environment and the properties of the various optomotor reactions involved. The latter may not be much more complicated than the sketches offered here.

Hierarchies of Motor Control

For certain motor tasks, a sufficiently high-level choice of strategy need not involve specification of the details of execution at the muscular level. For example, in writing a word, we use a completely different set of muscles, depending on whether the instrument available is a pencil or whether it is a paintbrush on the end of a long pole. How is it that we can still produce our characteristic mode of writing with these two different systems? Computer scientists find it expedient to program a computer not in the machine language that directly controls the basic operations of its machinery but rather in terms of some high-level language. They provide the computer with a supervisory program, called an "interpreter," that will enable the computer to translate each instruction from the high-level program and then execute it. Analogously, we might suggest that the brain accumulates high-level motor routines in terms of sequences of variously directed motions and in terms of relative position but without any specific reference to the absolute position in which, or the part of the body with which, those motions are to be effected. It might then be hypothesized that our learning has also built up an interpreter for these high-level routines, one for each of many different body systems. Thus, so long as the high-level program is available, any such system may execute fairly skilled movements even though it has never executed them before. This explanation seems to accord well with the example of writing with a pencil and a paintbrush. Of course, it still leaves open the fundamental question of what mechanisms may actually exist in the brain for abstracting high-level routines from skills learned solely with one system and for constructing interpreters for different systems. Also, there is the question of the extent to which it is really tenable to make a sharp distinction between high-level language, the interpreter, and the machine language of the effector systems themselves.

Feedforward and Feedback

The foregoing discussion suggests that we view complex motor activity as being performed by the piecing together of substructures, each dealing with limited aspects of the problem. An important task in building up brain theory, then, is to isolate the substructures of motor behavior and to investigate ways in which they are combined to produce coordinated actions. (See the extensive theoretical studies on this problem by Greene (1969, 1971, 1972, 1973a,b,d, 1975a,b); the experimental studies of the Russian school founded by N. Bernstein will be discussed in Chapter V.) To gain some feel for this composition problem, we may, as did Greene (1972), look at a visual display system designed by Dertouzos (1967; Dertouzos and Graham, 1966) to generate patterns by directing a beam of electrons in a cathode ray tube. Clearly, the most general approach is to describe a pattern by its brightness at every point on the screen. This way, all possible patterns can be displayed. A second method, which is much more efficient for most interesting patterns, is to piece together standard, parameterized curves. Dertouzos's display uses the second method (see Figure 6). By setting about four parameters to appropriate values by means of Inputs 2, a large family of curves can be traced when a "draw" command is issued. Next, one might add a subsystem that generates appropriate tuning inputs for a parameterized set of about ten standard curves. Inputs to a higher level controller would be the label of the particular curve, its orientation, time of initiation, initiation point, and size, which would be converted to appropriate tuning parameters for the curve generators. Such a system could begin to function like a draftsman's French curve.

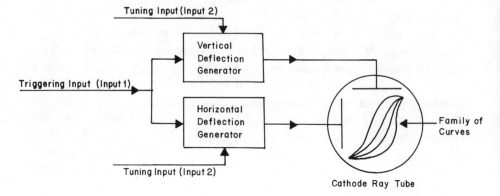

Figure 6. A triggering input causes a curve to be traced across the screen of the cathode ray tube; this curve can be modified via the tuning inputs to provide the family of curves shown in part here. [Greene]

In Greene's (1972) *theory of tasks*, the crucial principle is the separation of responsibility for activation and tuning. *Activating* the right *function generator* for a movement may be caricatured as "getting into the right ball park," whereas *tuning* the action to current circumstances requires adjusting within the "ball park." Thus, in the preceding example, a ball park could be a parameterized family of curves (Figure 7) produced by a particular tunable function generator.

A classic example of this separation of responsibility is as follows: when a cat prepares to pounce, before the movement itself is released, the orientation of the cat's head and body and the tension in its muscles are so adjusted that, when the pounce is actually made, it ends precisely on the mouse. It seems reasonable to suggest that the

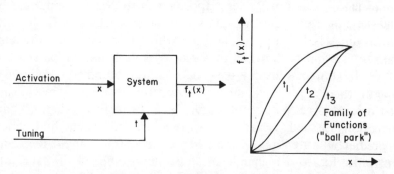

Figure 7. In the general organization shown in Figure 6, a system is activated and tuned by inputs (*x* and *t*, respectively) that are produced relatively independently. In this way, a standardized activating input, *x*, can result in any one of a family of output functions, $f_t(x)$. This family of functions is a "ball park" in the sense that any one of its members may be converted into any other by tuning, with which the activating system need not be concerned. [Greene]

"executive" releases the movement independent of the actual target position, but that the motor system is already tuned beforehand through external parameters, such as the position of the mouse. Boylls's model for the cerebellum (see Chapter V) employs this strategy.

Control by means of ball park and tuning mechanisms results in the system's having certain properties such as the following: (1) There is ambiguity in that the executive is unaware of the tuning and therefore does not distinguish which curve in the family of curves has been generated. (2) Different generators are needed in various ranges, as in the case of differing speed/foot-pedal-angle relations of a car being driven in different gears. The low-level controller knows the "set" of generators whose functions coincide over the range of action: low-level detectors can be used to select the appropriate function in this equivalence class. (3) "Patch-up" circuitry is then required to handle transitions from one region to another (cf. the transition from one gait to another). Many different generators can thus seem equivalent to the executive. Boylls, however, suggested that equivalence classes are too rigid if energy considerations are ignored, and he noted the relevance of the Russian "principle of least interaction," i.e., that an efficient system has minimal interaction of its subsystems with each other and with the environment (Gelfand et al., 1971, pp. 16-20), to the self-organization of interactions between function generators (see pp. 157-165).

There are also sensory examples; for example, the slide box idea of an internal model is based on this, the slides providing the ball-park selection of actions that are then tuned by the fine details of sensory input. The notion of an output feature cluster was designed to suggest how reducing the degrees of freedom in the input may provide access to motor synergies appropriate for interaction with the current environment.

It should be noted that none of the conventional notions of control theory is discarded in this scheme. Feedback and perhaps feedforward (i.e., using input information to compute responses and corrections rather than waiting for feedback, or, perhaps, using a model to predict what is about to happen) are used to implement each local controller. Exactly what is being gained by the use of feedforward and by the separation of responsibility into ball-park and fine-tuning systems cannot be quantified until the nature of the computation is better understood, and an appropriate theory of computation complexity developed; but the goal is to reduce the computation required at high levels at the expense of more local, less general, more autonomous, simpler controllers. This suggests that we consider the two types of feedforward discussed below. We shall then discuss the better known process of feedback, which serves to reduce the complexity of a controller that must compensate for unanticipated disturbances.

Feedforward as a Function of Input

If control is solely by feedforward mechanisms, then it must be extremely precise. Generally, gross feedforward is used to bring the system into the correct ball park and, then, simple feedback can correct for any further errors. When feedforward is applied to a complex system, the complexity of control is reduced because the system is kept within a ball-park region of the operation. As a result, feedback is applied to a resultant, much simpler system. However, feedback alone may yield unsatisfactory control because of the time lag. For example, if we want to maintain constant output composition from an oil distillation column, the time lag involved in the passage of material through the column would cause oscillations for a simple feedback system. However, feedforward, even if based on as gross a model as a second-order model of a distillation column, can restore reasonable stability of the system. For a cat balancing on a tilted platform, a rough feedforward based on vestibular input is required for the cat to maintain its posture, keeping activity in the "domain of attraction" where feedback can independently use muscle spindle information to "tune" each leg—feedback is of little use to an animal sprawled upside down. Of course, when the executive issues an "override," the subordinate system must not try to compensate for it, as when head turning cancels the vestibular reflex.

Feedforward That Disguises a Complex System

In this case, feedforward is used to alter a complex system continuously so that its behavior always conforms to that of some simple model system and is thus controllable by uniform strategies, as in the "model-reference" control of an airplane shown in Figure 8 (Whitaker, 1962, 1963; Dressler, 1967; Porter, 1969). Inputs applied to this apparently simple system can then be used for control. Note, however, that one cannot make an arbitrary airplane behave like an arbitrary model; in other words, the model system selected must be in the right ball park of model systems. (In Chapter V, Ito's (1972a,b, 1974) idea on feedforward in vestibular-cerebellar interactions will be discussed.)

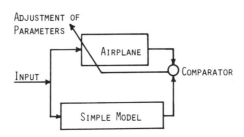

Figure 8. The pilot's control signals are fed to a simple model as well as to the otherwise unmanageable airplane, and the differences between the responses of the two are used to compute the adjustment of parameters of the airplane that make it respond more like the simple model. [Greene]

Simplification is often achieved by restricting the degrees of freedom of the original system. Since it is difficult to control independently all the degrees of freedom in a system, it may be desirable to lump some of them or make them change together, e.g., make muscles into functional groups. However, this lumping eliminates many possible movements and thus restricts the universe of the system's possible behavior. Forming "synergies" (according to the Russian terminology discussed in Chapter V) further excludes certain types of movements while simplifying the control of other types, but it may be good enough to approximate what you usually want to do.

Feedback in Spinal Control of Movement

Turning to the role of feedback in the spinal control of movement, we note that the α-motoneuron system can quickly elicit an approximately correct response, while feedback "follow up" by the γ-motoneuron system frees the other parts of the nervous system from having to involve slight variations in peripheral conditions in their computations (Evarts et al., 1971). It is tempting to regard the α-motoneuron system as providing the ballistic component and the γ-motoneuron system as superposing a tracking component in a mixed ballistic-tracking strategy, which gets the system into new states quickly without losing the benefits of feedback compensation.

With these considerations, the joint virtue of hierarchical organization and of local feedback to "reduce the burden of computation on higher levels" is obvious. The examination of circuitry could continue, showing the following: (1) how the neurons controlling the various joints of a single limb are interrelated, (2) how the two limbs of a single pair are related by what are called *intrasegmental reflexes*

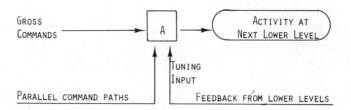

Figure 9. A generalization of the schemes shown in Figures 6 and 7. Feedback from lower levels in an animal motor system and parallel command paths provide tuning inputs for the movements triggered by gross commands. [Modified from Arbib, 1972a]

because they occur within a single segment of the spinal cord, and (3) how these are utilized in the *intersegmental reflexes,* which unite various segments of the spinal cord in smoothly controlling automatic postural adjustments and the sequence of stepping in locomotion.

For the animal motor system, the schemes of Figures 6 and 7 would be redrawn as shown in Figure 9. Here, at any stage in the hierarchy, the actions taken are dependent upon a gross command, which is tuned mainly by measurements of local conditions in adjacent levels. The gross commands need only be "in the right ball park," i.e., close enough to the desired trajectory so that the abilities of the tuning inputs to correct are not exceeded. A good example is the notion of a postural frame within which movements take place. Lower-level feedback via spinal reflexes can serve to keep an animal from falling over despite changing support conditions. Commands to move need not carry information about what will happen to the center of gravity if a certain leg is lifted—the postural tuning inputs will cause the whole body (if necessary) to move so as to provide proper support. Parallel command paths can then impose refinements (such as the finger movements involved in playing the piano) on the gross trajectory with feedback stabilization. (The reader may wish to relate these comments to the discussion on "Corollary Discharge" above.)

Much motor control is hierarchical in the sense that groups of motor neurons, rather than individuals, are patterned. Further, much of the outflow consists of predictions of what these groups of effectors will do. This outflow goes to relatively high spinal centers and is checked against feedback from lower regions and the periphery. These "correlation centers" can then "report" to the cerebrum on the extent to which movements are "progressing as planned." (This postulation is similar to the idea of internal feedback of Evarts and his colleagues (1971).) Each central pattern for the initiation of movement has its neuronal repercussions upon central sensory patterns, and each performed movement introduces alterations in sensory input patterns. In this way, sensory and motor systems are bound together both internally and externally.

Minimal Structural Requirements of Coordinated Movement

Theoretically, a single neuron or very few (i.e., 2 to 4), mutually interconnected neurons might well be capable of containing whole programs of complex command sequences, which they might execute either with the aid of motoneurons or even without such aid if they have direct connections to muscles. There are numerous examples of this in the nervous system of invertebrates. Although it is quite conceivable that such neurons are present in vertebrates, the clear differences between the motor output of nonorganoid cell assemblies of medullary tube origin (discussed in Chapter III) and those of clearly organoid nature (also treated in Chapter III) would point in another direction. It seems, rather, that the neural organization of vertebrates has adopted another strategy, namely, to rely on neuronal networks rather than on single, specific types of neurons (the so-called "unique neurons") for encoding and decoding messages as well as programs.* This does not imply that the possible existence of unique neurons is categorically rejected for the vertebrates. The widespread notion among neuroscientists that there should be a fundamental difference between the neural organization of invertebrates and vertebrates with respect to the occurrence or nonoccurrence of unique neurons has been only recently attacked with convincing arguments (Bullock, 1974). It is, a priori, certainly possible that, eventually, a few unique "master neurons" containing the programs for walking patterns in the limb segments of the medullary tube will be found. But this is extremely unlikely in view of the experimental embryological facts (discussed in Chapter III) and especially in regard to the finding that even a part of any one of the limb segments of the medullary tube appears to contain the whole basic program for walking or for other specific limb movement patterns (Weiss, 1950b), for example, the complex wing movement patterns of birds triggered by vestibular reflexes (Straznicky,

*This strategy seems reasonable, or understandable, in view of the fact that limitations upon an increase in the number of neurons are far less stringent in vertebrates than in most invertebrates. However, when we go from molluscs to invertebrates that have layered nervous systems, such as flies and octopuses, the separation begins to blur.

1963). Otherwise, we would have to assume that each of the limb segments has to contain a number of such master neurons, and, thus, we would essentially be back to the concept we started with (see p. 66 in Chapter III): the basic programs for walking patterns are contained in a number of specifically interconnected, interneuronal discs or chips (see Figure 15 in Chapter III). This would then be the minimal requirement in neuronal organization for coordinated movement.

Complexity and Hierarchies

It is worth noting that certain behaviors that might be complicated to simulate on a computer may be very simple properties of the nervous system and body. Because of gravity, it requires no detailed computation to put one's arm down. Again, the relationship between the shape of the limbs and the function that they are to subserve affects requirements for neural computation. Much work is being done by anatomists, and especially those interested in evolution, to understand how a change in the structure of the skeleton correlates with a change of function. Presumably, there are many different ways one could put joints together and get a system that could carry out certain manipulations. For some structures these will be easy manipulations to control, whereas for others, control will be difficult. Automata theory offers theorems about how changes in input coding can drastically change the amount of time a network would take to carry out a computation (Bobrow and Arbib, 1974). For any given function, there seems to be a best way of coding the information to get a fast response from the system. Similarly, the way in which we structure the musculature and the bones will greatly affect the amount of computation that is required to assure a smooth operation of joints and easy interaction of the organism with the world. Thus, an "old-fashioned" part of mechanical engineering—the study of kinematic linkages—may, as Greene has suggested, become increasingly relevant to us; it can augment our studies of pure information processing and tell us how to put bars and rods together, and put joints between them, so that the resultant motions of the linkage describe an appropriate curve without having to be "pushed" by elaborate computation through each successive point of its orbit. For example, the "simple" function $y = x$ and the "complex" function $y = \log \tan (x \log x)$ are equally easy to generate mechanically; both are done by linking bars of different lengths so that the arm moves appropriately. The linkages reduce the degrees of freedom, thus permitting only one family of functions, while tuning can be obtained by adjusting the lengths of the bars. Computational tasks depend not only upon input preprocessing but also upon the output structures that actually execute the actions.

III. A STRUCTURAL OVERVIEW

Whereas we attempted in Chapter II to outline the principal logical and functional requirements that have to be met (by nature) to produce a command and control system like the brain, in this chapter we assess the structural organization of neural systems and how this might serve the outlined requirements. In Chapter II the logic of our reporting was to proceed from the "top down" as we tried to understand what kind of organization would be needed to make all the detailed multilevel computations and decisions to weld the often-conflicting reflex and lower behavioral mechanisms into the purposefully behaving whole of the individual. In this chapter, conversely, we proceed from the "bottom up," taking account of the various kinds of neuronal machinery available at the several levels, and of how they might be put together in hierarchical (or other) orders to meet the principal requirements, as far as we can understand them today.

Neural Networks

It is appropriate to begin this section by considering the neuroanatomical data on neural networks, particularly the importance of the geometry and orientation of the dendritic and axonal arborizations. These orderly patterns of arborization introduce organization into networks even when there appears to be random synaptic contact by an axon with every dendrite it encounters. Even in random networks without orderly arborizations, extremely organized patterns of electrical activity are generated. This is discussed in terms of the deplantation experiments on newt limbs and the available .theoretical models of random neural nets.

The concept of neural nets entered the thinking of neuroscientists at a relatively early stage (around the middle of the nineteenth century) when the long processes of the nerve cells and their intricate mutual intertwinement became known (Gerlach, 1872). Later, this became the main battlefield of the "reticularists," and the expression "neural or neuronal net" was still suspect for many neuroscientists until the turn of the century, when the neuron bècame accepted as the basic cellular element of neural tissue and as its anatomical, developmental (genetic), functional, trophic, and pathological unit. We now know that neural tissues, despite their being built of independent cellular units joined together in specific ways and at specific sites (i.e., the synapses), are much less sequential chains than they are networks of intricately interconnected neurons. Sequential connections do exist, but less between individual neurons than between different groups of neurons that are connected by a number of parallel channels.

The original idea of the neuron network as a continuum of nerve cells of standard shape(s) and isotropic (random or geometrically determined) connectivity properties has all but disappeared from our image of the centers of the higher animals; however, it may still hold in our knowledge of the primitive neural nets in some, but only some, invertebrates such as the coelenterates (Bullock and Horridge, 1965). The obvious advantages of such networks have been exploited by theoreticians (Beurle, 1954; Farley, 1964) and modelers (Reiss, 1964). The model of Wilson and Cowan (1972), to be discussed in Chapter IV, is very much in the Beurle tradition, but it introduces enough extra structure to make its heuristic significance for the neurosciences less questionable.

A certain revival in the consideration of the network aspects of neural tissue structure can be recognized, under radically changed conditions, in recent trends in neuroanatomy (Colonnier, 1966; Szentágothai, 1964a,b,c, 1965, 1967a,b; Scheibel and Scheibel, 1958, 1966, 1969). Ramón y Cajal's (1909, 1911) diagrams, particularly on cerebellar cortex, hippocampus, tectum, retina, olfactory bulb, etc., bear witness to his ingenious insights into the organizational principle of neuron networks. Furthermore, one should not forget that the apparently diffuse appearance of certain networks could be simply due to our failure to grasp a three-dimensional organization that does not manifest itself in the form of clear-cut clusters, layers, or columns of nerve cells (Ramón-Moliner and Nauta, 1966). In spite of these insights, the limited knowledge at Ramón y Cajal's time about the function of individual neurons and synapses did not permit any significant progress along these lines until the elegant speculations, based on anatomical observations, of Lorente de Nó (1922, 1932, 1933, 1938) on two major principles of neuron coupling: the "multiplicity" and "reciprocity" of neural connections. Undoubtedly, it is here that reasoning about elementary neural functions in terms of simple neuron networks (not necessarily confined to any restricted piece of gray matter) has its modern origin. (The "association" psychologists of the nineteenth century made great use of hypothetical neural networks, but these were not based on any real neuroanatomy.) Lorente de Nó's speculations (1933, 1938) on "delay lines" and "reverberating circuits" in terms of simple neuron-coupling models offered the first rational explanation of the basic functional events, beyond those happening on the level of a single synapse, that may account for the integrative function in neural structures. This, again, remained a blind alley until the discovery of specific inhibitory interneurons (Eccles et al., 1954a,b) in two spinal reflex mechanisms opened the way for new concepts and our present understanding of neuron networks.

It then became unavoidable that, in various known specific neuron networks, excitatory and inhibitory roles be assigned to the various neuron types, at first arbitrarily and, later, on the basis of direct physiological evidence. In the cerebellar cortex, such a speculative approach (Szentágothai, 1963a, 1965) led to apparently meaningful results that could be tested directly by physiological experiments (Eccles, 1965) and led eventually to the concept of the neuron network as a "specific neuron machine" (Eccles et al., 1967).

A similar approach is presently being developed for the "neuron machine" of the neocortex, although this is still in the early stages of speculation based on anatomical structure (Szentágothai, 1967a, 1969, 1971, 1972a). Any further development will depend on direct physiological experiments specifically designed to test, i.e., to prove or to disprove, the anatomical predictions. The visual system served as one of the major models in the search for the principles of neocortical neural organization, and its circuit model will be considered in more detail in a later section.

Neural Network: A Continuum or Separable Units?

To what extent should a neural network be considered as a continuum or, conversely, how far can it be subdivided into separable functional units? The efforts of the cytoarchitectonic schools (Vogt, 1903; Vogt and Vogt, 1919; Economo and Koskinas, 1925; Rose, 1935) to subdivide the cerebral cortex into sharply delineated small regions—almost into different organs—were an expression of the feeling that what is essentially (or apparently) a continuum ought to be subdivided into smaller discrete units. The same problem arises in a somewhat different form for the "pathway neuroanatomist," who traces connections by means of degeneration, and to whom the subdivision of any piece of gray matter is often determined, consonant with Principle 5 of Chapter II, by the somatotopic arrangement* within the projection of either afferent or efferent pathways.

The possibility of a much finer subdivision of apparently continuous neural gray matter than the most radical cytoarchitectonicist could ever have dreamt of is suggested by the columnar arrangement of receptive field projections in sensory cortices (Mountcastle, 1957; Hubel and Wiesel, 1962, 1963, 1965). Following up this lead, as well as certain experimental embryological observations on the spinal segmental apparatus and a logical consideration of the neuronal machine of the cerebellar cortex, Szentágothai (1967a) attempted to subdivide apparently continuous bulks of gray matter into pieces of minimal size that, on the basis of their preserved original internal connectivity, could still be considered essentially the same as the neuronal machine and be capable of the same elementary tasks of information processing as the whole. Such theoretically assumed minimum-sized pieces of neuron networks were labeled "integrative units" of the neural tissue.

The reality of such larger units had been tested experimentally only in the embryonic spinal cord (see below); however, the concept has recently received strong support from the observation of the so-called "cortical barrels" (Woolsey and Van der Loos, 1970) to be discussed below. Generally, the concept of a modular organization of nerve networks, or specifically, of the neuropil has been current for some time and will also be discussed from various viewpoints below.

"Randomness" Versus Specificity of Structure

When looking at any piece of central nervous tissue, the beholder is immediately aware of two conflicting aspects and interpretations of structure. On the one hand, the long dendritic arborizations and their frequent intertwinement with widespread, highly irregular and diffuse terminal axon arborizations would suggest a random connectivity between the several pre- and postsynaptic elements participating in any piece of neuropil. This is particularly striking in the brainstem

---

*The major exponents of this important direction of inquiry into the finer spatial arrangements of neural projection are A. Brodal and the neuroanatomy investigators at the University of Oslo.

reticular formation (isodendritic core) as pointed out by Ramón-Moliner and Nauta (1966). On the other hand, investigations with the classical Golgi method, reinforced by the recent possibility of tracing connections at the ultrastructural level, seem to indicate that there is an extremely strict specificity, not only with respect to what kind of neuron is contacted by any given type of axon but also concerning the exact site where the synapse is established (cell body, proximal and distal part of the dendrite, dendrite surface proper or dendritic spine, etc.).

Thus, in this section the term "randomness" should not be taken literally for the following reasons: first, because what might appear as random to the uninitiate might contain in reality a rather specific design (as is, in fact, the case with computer wiring); second, although connections may be restricted only statistically and the position of the individual contact may be completely undesigned, it cannot be labeled as truly random. As used here, the word "random" should be understood as "undesigned" in the sense that its design is not *yet* clear to us.

A major attempt to deal quantitatively with apparently random connectivity in specific nerve nets was made by Sholl (1956), whose ingenious studies on dendritic arborizations led to certain general formulations that could be used to predict the probability* of contacts between any dendrite arbor and various types of terminal axonal arborizations coexistent in space with the former (Uttley, 1956). However, in order for this kind of an approach to lead to a better understanding of the connectivity in neuron networks, both the dendritic and axonal arborization patterns needed clarification. In the cerebral cortex, for example, the terms "pyramidal neuron" and "stellate neuron" are rather uninformative. An important step forward in this direction was made by Ramón-Moliner and Nauta (1966) who attempted to establish a general classification of the nerve cells of the brainstem that, for the first time, tried to correlate dendritic morphology and neuronal function. Their classification principle (shown in Figure 10) emphasizes the presence of a numerous class of generalized ("isodendritic") nerve cells that correspond partially to what was earlier labeled, rather indiscriminately, as "stellate." It does not deal with cell types having highly specific and/or polarized dendritic arborizations (like the pyramidal cells of the cerebral or the Purkinje cells of the

*Since a specific scheme of connections may still lend itself to useful statistical descriptions, Sholl's results do not preclude cortical specificity.

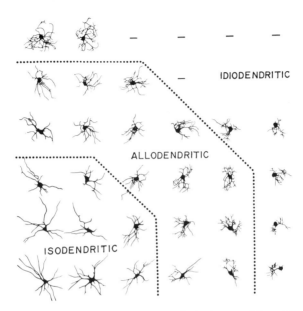

Figure 10. Varieties of dendritic patterns found in the brainstem of the cat. The cells with the most generalized or isodendritic arborization patterns are shown in the lower left corner. Progressive specialization proceeds from the allodendritic neurons towards the most specialized idiodendritic cell types as indicated in the respective zones. Specialization in the idiodendritic cell type may proceed towards waviness (upwards in the vertical direction) or towards tuftedness (horizontally to the right) of the dendritic tree. [Ramón-Moliner and Nauta, 1966]

cerebellar cortex, or the numerous other cells in the hippocampus, olfactory bulb, etc.), which might be considered simply as extreme (and even more specific) forms of their "idiodendritic" type.

This classification is essentially based on: (1) "randomness" versus "regularity" in regard to branching of the various dendritic segments (in site, sequence, length, and number), resulting in a graded morphological spectrum ranging from the "radiate" to the "tufted" types of arborization; and (2) the degree of deviation of the individual branches from a basically radiated and rectilinear course. The "wavy" and, in its extreme degree, "recurving" (see Figure 10) character of the dendrites would, obviously, radically change the equations established by Sholl (1956) for the number of dendrites piercing the concentric spherical shells envisaged around the centers of the cell bodies (Figure 11). The density of dendritic intersections would be larger in the wavy and considerably larger in the recurving type of dendrite arborizations (other parameters being equal) than in straight radial arborizations. Similarly, in the tufted dendritic trees, the density of intersections would be relatively higher in the outer shells than has been

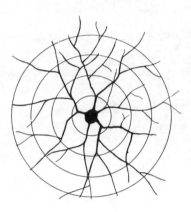

Figure 11. The method designed by Sholl for describing dendritic arborizations in quantitative terms. Concentric spherical shells, with radii increasing in equal steps, are imagined to be arranged around the center of the soma; the number of dendritic branches piercing each of the shell spheres is then counted. [Sholl, 1953]

established for ordinary radial arborizations. However, on the assumption of identical parameters for the length of the dendritic segments, the number of intersections would fall off more steeply in the outer spherical shells. In addition, the external radius of the sphere containing the entire dendritic arborization would be reduced in the cell types with wavy or tufted types, and would be radically smaller in those having recurving dendrites. The original reasonings of Ramón-Moliner and Nauta (1966) were applied to the brainstem neurons only; the strongly "polarized" or "nonspheric" dendritic trees (e.g., spindle-shaped, "cellules à double bouquet" of Ramón y Cajal, and disc-shaped) were not considered. However, these arguments could also apply to them with certain restrictions (see Ramón-Moliner, 1967, 1968, 1970).

At any rate, either the wavy or recurving character increases the compactness of the arborization, i.e., the fraction of dendrite volume in the unit volume of the total space occupied by the dendrite arborization (which is equal to the density of dendrite volume in total neuropil space). This is, of course, obvious and almost trivial, but it is of crucial importance if one is to appreciate fully the significance of the classification of Ramón-Moliner and Nauta (1966) for synaptic connectivity.

Again, other parameters (number of primary, secondary, etc., dendritic branches and total dendritic length) being equal, the restriction (in volume fraction) of the dendrites of any given neuron to its own neuropil is smallest in the isodendritic, higher in the allodendritic, and highest in the idiodendritic cell category. Consequently, since there is practically no empty space in the neuropil, the following conclusions can be made: (1) the dendrites of relatively distant cells are more likely to mingle in the case of the general or isodendritic neuron; (2) in the neuropil of nerve centers or regions populated by isodendritic cells, more synapses between the dendrites of a given nerve cell and branches of different axons are likely to be established (assuming that the axonal arborizations participating in the neuropil have the same geometric and topologic features); (3) in the allodendritic and, increasingly, in the idiodendritic cell-type neuropil, there will be more synaptic contacts established between any given cell and the branches of fewer axons. In other words, until proof to the contrary is obtained, in a neuropil containing cells with arborizations of the isodendritic type, the connectivity could be *more randomlike,* whereas in the allodendritic and, particularly, the idiodendritic neuropils, it will be circumscribed to fewer axonal arborizations and, hence, *more specific.* It is necessary, though, to stress that this reasoning applies only to the general cell type originally called stellate, i.e., cells having an isotropic dendritic tree of essentially spherical shape. Whenever the dendritic tree is polarized (for example, fusiform), the axis orientation of the neuropil elements (discussed below) becomes more important, imposing limitations on these general principles. The speculations about nerve cell arborization of several authors have been gradually moving in this direction (Bodian, 1952; Scheibel and Scheibel, 1958; Leontovich and Zhukova, 1963; Szentágothai, 1952a, 1966). However, it was the elegant concept of Ramón-Moliner and Nauta (1966) that gave clearer direction to such speculations (Szentágothai, 1967b, 1968, 1969, 1971).

Although a general theory of nerve-process arborization and neuropil geometry is still sorely lacking, specific elements have been available for several years and should be briefly mentioned here. Some of these elements are seen in the work of Uttley (1956) on the probability of geometric connections between interlacing arborizations. Others come from a general concept taking shape gradually: the modular structure of the neuropil, as exemplified in the "poker chip" model that Kilmer and his co-workers (1969) based on the anatomical work of Scheibel and Scheibel (1958). These elements will be discussed in the next sections by considering the following: first, the possibility of a completely random or undesigned connectivity between irregular dendritic and axonal arborizations; second, the significance of a specific axis orientation of the interlacing dendritic and axonal arborizations; and, finally, the modular concept itself.

Random or Quasi-Random Neural Networks

More or less random neuron networks can be artificially created by tissue culturing. It is well known from recent studies (Bunge and Bunge, 1965; Murray, 1965; Crain, 1973a,b) that new synapses can develop in tissue cultures and that electrophysiological signs of impulse transmission appear simultaneously with their development. It might be a matter of argument as to what extent such neuron networks really have a random connectivity, since even completely segregated neuron populations tend to reaggregate eventually in quasi-organoid patterns (Sidman, 1974) and appear to develop neuropil organization similar to that of normal brain centers. On the other hand, there is no evidence from tissue culture material of any specific neurotropic attraction between certain types of neurons or between neurons and the tissues they normally innervate, at least beyond the rather nonspecific mechanisms elucidated in the classical studies of Weiss (1950b). For example, there is no evidence that prospective motoneurons would grow more readily into muscle than any other neuron. (From this point of view it is entirely immaterial that striated muscle can be innervated functionally by prospective motoneurons exclusively.)

The deplantation technique, developed by Weiss (1950a) in larval newts, offers certain advantages for the study of nerve tissue fragments deplanted into the dorsal fin of larval hosts. This is so in that it is easy to let deplanted tissue innervate a larval limb implanted nearby, and also because reaggregation is less likely to occur in the more rigidly structured environment. Thus, the experimenter can intentionally produce more or less organoid deplants simply by deplanting neural organ fragments gently, without disruption of the original interrelations of the elements, or, conversely, by deplanting the early larval tissue as a disrupted mash. As was shown earlier by Weiss (1950a), but more specifically by Székely and Szentágothai (1962) and Székely and Czéh (1971a,b), both kinds of deplants can successfully (and with clear functional results) innervate the limb deplanted into the neighborhood. However, while the limb movements may retain unmistakable traces of the normal walking pattern whenever the deplanted cord tissue shows clear organoid structure and has been taken from the segments of the medullary tube that normally innervate limbs (Székely and Czéh, 1971a,b), nothing of this can be recognized if either the deplant has lost its organoid structure or if it is taken from any other part of the spinal cord or the lower brainstem, however well preserved the organoid character might otherwise be.

As shown by Székely and Szentágothai (1962), as few as 15 preserved neurons (of which only 3 to 4 appeared to be motoneurons), completely scattered and without the remotest resemblance to any organoid structure, can produce the distinctive movement pattern described by Weiss (1950a). The limb moves in a completely "epileptoid" manner, with different preparations showing different characteristics. Strychnine effects could also be readily demonstrated in the complete absence of any primary sensory elements. The conclusion reached at that time was that the deplants apparently contained a few excitatory and inhibitory interneurons, the random connections and the spontaneous activity of which would secure the motor activity over the few motoneurons that had successfully innervated the muscles of the limb. In spite of the irregularity and virtual unpredictability of the detailed activity of these deplants, Székely and Szentágothai (1962) were impressed by the relative order prevailing in a large number of deplants consisting of 10 to 20 to several hundreds or even thousands of neurons, the movement patterns of which did not seem to correlate significantly with the size of the deplant. They interpreted this as being the result of "self-organizing tendencies" in the function of these random or quasi-random networks.

It is interesting to note how this behavior of supposedly randomly interconnected populations of excitatory and inhibitory interneurons was predicted a posteriori by theoretical studies (Legéndy, 1967; Anninos et al., 1970; Harth et al., 1970; Wilson and Cowan, 1972) that analyzed the behavior of such neuron populations by a kind of statistical mechanics (see a more detailed discussion of the Wilson-Cowan study in Chapter IV).* While it is granted that the histology of these deplants looks random, it does not, in fact, prove that the connections between the surviving neurons are, indeed, so. However, the theoretical analysis of the behavior of networks of randomly interconnected excitatory and inhibitory interneurons shows that, if the interconnections were random in the deplanted tissue fragments, they would exhibit some of the observed characteristics. It is

---

*Note, too, the general observation that random nets have limit cycles; see especially the work of Kauffman (1970a).

a challenge to the theorist to face the detailed results of the deplantation experiments, though the experiments have not yielded all the parameters required for such analysis.

Significance in Neuron Nets of the General Orientation of Neuropil Elements

One major geometric factor determining connectivity in the neuropil (in Sholl's (1956) sense of the statistical probability of connection established between any two axonal and dendritic elements present in the same finite space) is the relative orientation of the dendrites to that of the axonal arborizations with which they are intertwined. In many cases this is random, or apparently so, with certain spatial restrictions, as, for example, if the neuropil is subdivided into smaller modules (as will be discussed later). However, it is often observed that the individual dendrites (or the dendritic tree as a whole) have a specific orientation relative to the predominant direction of the terminal axon branches (Ramón-Moliner, 1962). This aspect of neuropil architectonics has already received some theoretical consideration (Uttley, 1956); but it gained further significance from the recognition that consequences for synaptic connectivity are radically different according to whether the axons are intertwined with the dendrites at right angles to one another or are more or less aligned in parallel. The best example of the first case is the "crossing-over" synaptic arrangement in the parallel fiber-Purkinje cell synaptic system in the cerebellar cortex (Hámori and Szentágothai, 1964). The zonal layer of the cerebral cortex (Szentágothai, 1971) or the substantia gelatinosa (Szentágothai, 1964b) are further examples of such "crossing-at-right-angle" synaptic systems. The parallel alignment of an axonal and dendritic arborization is best exemplified by the climbing fibers of the cerebellum. Similar parallel alignments may also occur in the case of spiny dendrites, leading to the "rope ladder" phenomenon, stressed mainly by the Russian Golgi investigators (Poljakov, 1953; Shkolnik-Yarros, 1963).

The connectivity consequences of these two diametrically opposed arrangements are obvious: in a crossing-over arrangement the number of contacts (and hence the sum of contact surfaces) between any two given pre- and postsynaptic elements is close to one, whereas in the parallel alignment the number of contacts between any pair of synapsing elements may be on the order of hundreds or thousands (as in the case of cerebellar climbing fiber). Assuming that the total sum of postsynaptic sites in most neurons is within a certain range, this would mean that the "convergence" in neuron coupling is very high in the crossing-over synaptic arrangement and very low (approaching 1:1) in the parallel alignment, as, for example, in the climbing fiber-Purkinje cell contact.

The functional consequences of this are also predictable and correspond to neurophysiological observations. While threshold activation might require a high spatial summation in a crossing-over system, the activation might be "obligatory" (or close to 100% probability) in a parallel alignment system, as had been first postulated in observations on Clarke's column (Szentágothai and Albert, 1955).

Rall's (1962, 1964) theoretical models of dendritic geometry should be applied in all speculations about the possible functional consequences of any type of synaptic connectivity for which the reduction of the dendritic tree to a so-called "equivalent cylinder" is a useful simplification. The quantitative assumptions of this restriction seem to be in fair agreement with anatomical observations on the size relations between parent dendrites and their branches. The functional consequences on the cell body membrane potential (or on that of the generation site of the propagated impulse) can be readily predicted from the relative distances, in terms of equivalent cylinder length of the dendrite and the position and timing of the delivery of excitatory and/or inhibitory impulses to the dendritic tree. By combining Rall's diagram on the significance of the distance of the site of excitation from the cell body for soma-membrane potential changes *with* the arrangement of neuropil and synapses contacting the elongated dendritic tree of the spinal motoneuron (see Figure 6 in Scheibel and Scheibel, 1969), one sees a crucial difference between the time course of excitatory postsynaptic potentials, depending on whether they are produced by presynaptic activity in a disc closer to or more remote from the position of the cell body (Figure 12). The recent observations on synaptic transmission from Ia afferents to motoneurons (Mendell and Henneman, 1971) are in very good agreement with the prediction of the Rall model. Obviously, the same reasoning applies to all types of crossing-over axodendritic arrangements, particularly if the presynaptic afferents are systematically arranged in a laminated manner, as, for example, in the hippocampus and probably in the zonal layer of the cerebral cortex. It is not known whether there is any systematic arrangement of surface parallel laminas in the molecular layer of the

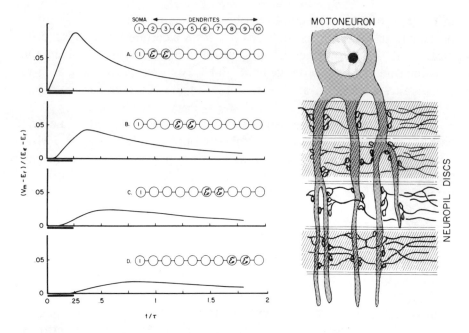

Figure 12. The assumed consequences in the spinal motoneuron of the arrangement of the axonal neuropil in transversally oriented layers as predicted by the dendritic model of Rall. Left figure shows the effect of excitatory ($\mathcal{E}$) pulse locations on transient soma-membrane depolarization. The soma-dendritic receptor surface is divided into ten equal compartments ($\Delta Z = 0.2$; where Z = electrotonic distance from the soma) as shown in top row. The four $\mathcal{E}$-pulse locations are shown in the diagrams beside the letters A, B, C, and D; in each case $\mathcal{E} = 1$ in two compartments for the time interval $0.25\ \tau$, indicated by the thick solid bars. These curves were drawn through computed value s for time steps of $0.05\ \tau$. To convert to real time, a τ value between 4 and 5 msec is appropriate. Right diagram shows the neuropil discs pierced successively by the longitudinal dendrites of motoneurons and containing a group of synapses that correspond to the ten compartments in A to D of the left figure. [Left figure, Rall, 1964; right diagram, Szentágothai]

cerebellar cortex such as we have tentatively hinted at (Eccles et al., 1967; see also Chapter V); if there is, it would be of great significance. The spatiotemporal sequence of impulses delivered to the same dendrite is of obvious importance in the parallel alignment type synapses, as occur between the climbing fiber and the Purkinje cell. Depending on the direction of the climbing contact and, hence, on the direction along the dendrite in which the impulses are successively delivered, the Rall model would predict the consequences for the soma-membrane potential as shown in Figure 13. The sequence is unequivocally cellulifugal in the climbing fiber-Purkinje cell synapse, whereas the direction may be more generally cellulipetal in Clarke's column and is

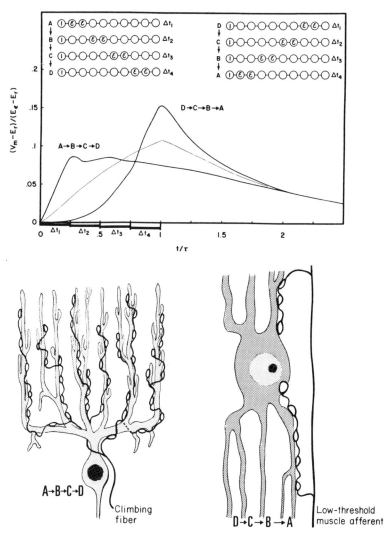

Figure 13. The assumed consequences (as predicted by the Rall model) of two spatiotemporal sequences on transient soma-membrane depolarization. The two $\mathscr{E}$-pulse sequences, A→B→C→D corresponding to the synaptic action of the cerebellar climbing fibers (lower left diagram) and D→C→B→A corresponding to the synaptic action of low-threshold muscle afferents in the Clarke neurons of the spinal cord (lower right diagram), are indicated in the top left-hand corner and top right-hand corner of upper figure. The component $\mathscr{E}$-pulse locations are the same as those in Figure 12. The time sequence is indicated by means of the four successive intervals, Δt_1, Δt_2, Δt_3, and Δt_4, each equal to $0.25\,\tau$. The magnitude, $\mathscr{E} = 1$, in the two compartments is the same as that in Figure 12. The dotted curve shows the computed effect of $\mathscr{E} = 0.25\,\tau$ in compartments 2 through 9 (see Figure 12) for a period $t = 0$ to $t = \tau$. [Upper figure, Rall, 1964; lower diagrams, Szentágothai and Albert, 1955]

probably generally cellulifugal in upper layers and cellulipetal in lower layers of the cerebral cortex, assuming that many of the Golgi type II cells giving rise to the majority of terminal axons that form parallel alignments (see below) are located in lamina IV. This becomes of great functional significance if the following possibilities are considered.

It is well known that the spatiotemporal dendritic simulation model of Rall (1964) could serve the function of simple detection of movement or frequency modulation. If the presynaptic afferents reaching a given neuron were arranged in a systematic fashion so that a change in stimulus pattern from the periphery could be conveyed to the dendritic tree in a spatiotemporal sequence, either away from or towards the cell body, the entirely different time course of the membrane potential change (Figure 13) could be used as a cue for the detection of the change of pattern and its direction. This mechanism would offer a parsimonious explanation of feature extraction and would account for the dependence of feature extraction on stimulus velocity (cf. Whitsel et al., 1972). However, it requires a precision of order in synaptic terminations that is difficult to conceive, let alone demonstrate with presently available methods. There are, however, situations in lower auditory centers where neurons specifically signal frequency modulation (Erulkar et al., 1968) and where the anatomical situation would entirely match the requirements of the mechanism (Harrison and Irving, 1966; Osen, 1969). If the anatomical situation were entirely as described by Harrison and Irving (1966) (see Figure 14), and the type k cells had only ascending dendrites, one would have to assume that all cells have the same direction of asymmetry in response to frequency modulation. However, since the "octopus cells" of Osen (corresponding to the type k cells of Harrison and Irving) can have either ascending or descending dendrites, embedded into the same frequency-laminated neuropil, an asymmetry in sensitivity may exist in both directions, as has been actually observed. Indeed, such functional consequences of neuropil geometry offer fascinating perspectives; however, it must be emphasized that these mechanisms would require an exceptionally high degree of order and would offer in exchange only extremely narrow ranges within which they could be effective. Therefore, it would be always unrealistic to look for similar "simple" geometric arrangements in our search for "feature extractors." It is more likely that feature extraction, even in such relatively simple cases as frequency modulation, relies on more sophisticated means (Suga, 1969).

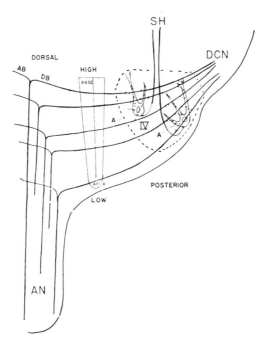

Figure 14. Tonotopic lamination of acoustic nerve terminals over the dendritic tree of Harrison's and Irving's (1966) type k neurons in region IV of the acoustic nucleus. Connections of the high-to-low frequency regions of the cochlea are indicated by the uncoiled cochlea superimposed on the nucleus. A indicates endings that do not arise from the acoustic nerve; AB = ascending branch, acoustic nerve; AN = acoustic nerve; DB = descending branch, acoustic nerve; DCN = dorsal cochlear nucleus; SH = stria of Held. [Harrison and Irving, 1966]

The same caution applies equally to cases where dendritic geometry can be assumed to be in some direct relationship with the spatial sensitivity of neurons; for example, in the retina the wide tangentially spread dendritic tree of the ganglion cells enables them to receive impulses from a considerable number of bipolar cells. This makes it possible to study the transfer properties of the retina in considerable detail (Creutzfeldt, 1970) and also to assign certain components of the transfer to certain synaptic layers or cell types. Neurons with wide dendritic spread, and which consequently receive large spatial convergence, could be, on the other hand, instrumental in the feature extraction operation of distinguishing large objects from small ones. The observations by Maturana and his co-workers (1960) on receptive field size versus dendritic tree diameter in the frog retina might clearly point in this direction. In fact, the cells are extremely widespread in the tectum of amphibians (Lázár and Székely, 1967), and perhaps even the category I cells in the lateral geniculate body (LGB) of the cat (Guillery, 1966) might also function in this way. Caution is advised, though, in adopting such simplistic geometric explanations except where, as is the case in the retina, the neurons receive an essentially homogeneous input at all dendritic branches. At higher levels, where each neuron receives a large variety of inputs of different origin at various points of its dendritic tree (e.g., Globus and Scheibel, 1967), assumptions of such straightforward isomorphisms between neural processing strategies and aims on the one hand and neural tissue structure and function on the other are at best questionable practices in the search for the basic principles of neural organization.

The Modular Structure of the Neuropil

The concept of a modular structure or arrangement of the neuropil has two basic sources: (1) a more indirect one from the notion that neuronal networks ought to be subdivided into distinct functional units and (2) a direct one from the observation of the neuropil. Functional and structural units resulting from the modular structure of the neuropil are explored in this section. The neuropil in the intermediate region and ventral horn of the spinal cord and in the reticular formation of the brainstem are discussed in terms of stacked "chips" of neuropil, with random interconnection within each chip but specific connectivity between chips. The cerebellar cortex also provides an elegant example of compartmentation of the neuropil and some new theoretical analyses are discussed. Recent anatomical data on the cerebral cortex suggest the existence of both a fine grain and a coarse grain modular organization in terms of slabs perpendicular to the cortical surface. Modular organization on a larger scale is exemplified by the "barrel" structure of the somatosensory cortex of the mouse. The successive stages or layers of processing in the cerebellar cortex or in the retinotectal system also constitute a modular organization where the spatial pattern of neural activity and its transformation at each stage are of interest.

Stacked Chips of Neuropil

The consideration of the spatial interrelations between dendritic and axonal arborizations was implicit in Ramón y Cajal's (1909, 1911) understanding of neuronal network structure. In his final summary and systematization (Ramón y Cajal, 1935), various types of synaptic arrangements and several specific concentrations of neuropil were enumerated (glomeruli of the olfactory bulb and the cerebellar cortex, dense nests of axonal arborizations encompassing a few or more postsynaptic perikarya, etc.), which correspond essentially to "modules." The first explicit statement, though, about a modular arrangement of the neuropil, including some discussion on its possible functional significance, was made by Scheibel and Scheibel (1958) in their description of the brainstem reticular formation. From their observation that both the dendritic arborizations of individual neurons and the terminal arborizations of individual axon collaterals, entering the reticular gray matter from the longitudinal fiber bundles, arborize in relatively narrow, transversally oriented discs, the Scheibels deduced their elegant model: the concept of the reticular formation as a series of disc-shaped modules stacked in perpendicular orientation to the brainstem axis. More recently, it turns out that this stacked chips arrangement of the neuropil holds even better for the intermediate region and the ventral horn of the spinal cord (Scheibel and Scheibel, 1969; Szentágothai and Réthelyi, 1973). However, the modular arrangement in the spinal cord differs significantly from that in the reticular formation as a consequence of the longitudinal orientation of the dendritic trees of the motoneurons, and thus numerous transversal neuropil discs can be pierced in succession, as shown in Figure 15. The possible significance of this in the light of Rall's (1962, 1964) concepts of dendritic geometry, as illustrated in Figure 12, has been considered by the Scheibels (1969). As already mentioned, this concept accords well with the conclusion by Mendell and Henneman (1971) on the significance of the size of the motoneuron in synaptic connectivity.

More important, perhaps, are considerations concerning the interneurons and their interconnections (recently reviewed in detail by Szentágothai and Réthelyi, 1973). The vast majority of the dendritic arborizations of spinal interneurons of the intermediate region and the ventral horn is confined to relatively narrow, transversally oriented disc-shaped space;* the geometric probability of any terminal axon branch coming into sufficiently close proximity with any dendrite branch is considerably greater (other parameters of the network being assumed equal) than in a network where orientations of both axons and

---

*M. Réthelyi, unpublished data.

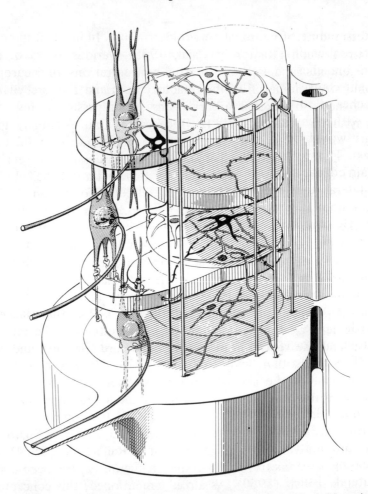

Figure 15. Stacked "chips" model of the spinal gray matter based on the ideas of Szentágothai (1967a), Scheibel and Scheibel (1969), and Szentágothai and Réthelyi (1973). The intermediate region can be considered as stacked disc-shaped chips containing excitatory (in outline) and inhibitory (solid) interneurons. The axonal neuropil of the ventral horn is arrayed in similar transversally oriented chips containing additional interneurons, from which only a single type, a Renshaw cell, is shown in the top chip. The motoneurons (stippled) pierce a number of successive ventral horn chips and receive synapses from each chip on the corresponding cylinder mantle of their soma or on the several cylinder mantles of their dendrites. Connectivity, particularly within the disc-shaped neuropil chips of the intermediate region, is assumed to be largely random or, at least, not strictly preaddressed. However, a rather high degree of order might be introduced into such a connectivity system by a set of "instructions" determining at what distances the longitudinally oriented axons of the several cell types have to issue collaterals to neighboring or more remote chips of the gray matter. It may be assumed on the basis of the observations of Székely and Czéh (1971a,b) on the functional capacities of isolated medullary tube segments that the minimal neuronal circuit capable of producing quasi-coordinated motor patterns would be something like that shown in this diagram. [Szentágothai]

dendrites are random in all the three dimensions of neuropil space. As has been emphasized earlier (Szentágothai, 1964c), the preterminal axon branches or collaterals cross the gray matter in remarkably straight courses (also illustrated in Figure 15), giving short terminal side branches at roughly equal distances. It has been argued on this basis that with such an arrangement it would be unreasonable to assume that axons would specifically seek contact with certain cells and avoid others. This situation is entirely different in the ventral horn, where certain collaterals both from primary (Ia) afferents and from the ventral and lateral funiculi are specifically directed to particular regions of the motor horn (Szentágothai, 1964c, 1967c) to establish contacts within narrowly confined territories, either on cell bodies or on the dendrites of the same or of closely neighboring motoneurons (Figure 15). In other words, a certain randomness (in the sense defined above) in the connectivity within the horizontal discs of the spinal intermediate region has to be assumed.

This randomness, however, is more apparent than real. Although the connectivity within the transversally oriented chips may be random, or nonaddressed, the connectivity between individual chips is not. This is apparent in many drawings of Ramón y Cajal (1909), who emphasized that collaterals from the ascending and descending main branches of the primary afferents, after their bifurcations in the dorsal funiculus, are issued to the gray matter not at random but at determined distances. The density of collateral branchings is greater in close proximity of the bifurcation and falls off progressively with increasing distance from the level of entrance into the cord. The collaterals issued by the same dorsal root also show characteristic changes with increasing segmental distance from the level of entrance, as shown by the early degeneration experiments of Schimert (1939). Even the collaterals of primary afferents, as, for example, the primary muscle spindle afferents (Ia), are of one kind at the level of their entrance and the two adjacent segments (in the lower lumbar and upper sacral cord); they become entirely different three to seven segments above their entrance where they are exclusively directed towards the Clarke nucleus (Szentágothai and Albert, 1955). The same holds true for both the medium-range intersegmental connections (Szentágothai, 1951) and for the more recently discovered short-range intrasegmental neurons (Mannen, 1969), whose axons send out transversally oriented preterminal collaterals (or branches) arborizing within transversal neuropil chips of the intermediate region and the ventral horn at apparently well-determined distances from the site of the cell body. The neuropil of the spinal gray matter (intermediate region and ventral horn) can thus be visualized as two parallel columns (for an earlier version of this, see Figure 4 of Szentágothai, 1967a) of stacked disc-shaped neuropil chips. The connections within any chip are virtually random (with the exception of the motoneurons), but those between chips (and those between any chip and the array of receptors at the periphery) are rather strictly patterned. Figure 15 tries to illustrate this with considerable simplification, completely neglecting the crossed connections between the two columns at both sides of the cord. As briefly indicated in a recent review paper (Réthelyi and Szentágothai, 1973), this general principle of characteristic types of collaterals occurring at determined distances from the segmental position of the cell body holds even better for the collaterals of crossed axons.

Expressed in other words, the example of the spinal cord might show how, by systematic stacking of modules of similar size and shape, "order in connectivity" can be established between the "disorderly built" modules simply by a "set of instructions" determining at what distances the axons, traveling along the stacks of modules, should issue their preterminal side branches. One might visualize the development of a rather highly specific internal connectivity of the spinal cord without a genetically predetermined program of what element has to connect with another;* a set of instructions for each type of cell, indicating at what distances (and at what times) collaterals ought to be issued from the ascending and descending branches of their axons, would suffice to bring about a highly specific connectivity structure.

The intermediate region of the spinal cord containing populations of excitatory and inhibitory interneurons could be envisaged metaphorically as a gearshift arrangement of a car (cf. Greene's (1969) views on regions of applicability of motor routines) or, more appropriately for this discussion, as an old-fashioned mechanical calculating machine in which cogwheels of various sizes mounted on a few parallel axles can produce a large variety of connections by shifting the axles back and forth into varying positions. The attractiveness of the modular concept illustrated in Figure 15 rests on the fact that very little specificity of connection would, obviously, be needed within the modules (in our metaphor a few cogwheels of different sizes would do);

---

*It is, of course, quite immaterial for this argument to indicate what causal chain prompts an axon to issue a collateral.

however, an enormous degree of specific interchangeability would be secured by the connections given to the modules by the various neurons participating in them.

Under normal circumstances, the characteristic "prewired" activities of the spinal segmental interneuron apparatus are triggered by descending commands from higher centers, and its functions are greatly modified by external feedback through afferent input. However, the spinal interneuron apparatus can obviously be triggered by the spontaneous activity of some of its own neurons, and, when once brought to activity, the network produces a built-in pattern. It remains conjectural how much, if any, of these built-in programs are retained in the spinal segmental apparatus of higher mammals. From clinical observations on rehabilitation of functions of the disconnected spinal cord, it seems reasonable to assume that much of the built-in central patterning of the spinal neuron network is retained and can be put to useful work even in man.

According to a host of experimental embryological experiments in urodeles and the chick, the programs for specific movement patterns are built into the segmental apparatus of the medullary tube. Brachial segments that are shifted to any site along the length of the medullary tube can innervate and move a forelimb (or wing in the chick) in the appropriate walking (or fluttering) pattern. Lumbosacral segments can do the same within a hindlimb (or leg in the chick) if shifted to any place along the axis of the cord. Recently, Czéh and Székely (1971) showed that medullary tube segments freely deplanted into the dorsal fin of newts (according to the technique developed by Weiss, 1950a), and innervating a simultaneously deplanted limb, can move this limb even in the absence of any connection with the CNS of the host and in the absence of spinal ganglia. They could show, by multichannel electromyographic recording from several muscles of the implanted limb, that the deplant produced bursts of rhythmic activity, resulting in recognizable "walking-type" movements of the deplanted limb. In order to obtain this result, two conditions were essential: (1) the segments had to be taken from either the brachial or the lumbar (i.e., the true) limb segments of the medullary tube, and (2) the deplant had to have a well-preserved organoid structure, i.e., a recognizable central canal with a surrounding well-developed intermediate zone and a differentiated ventral horn. The preservation of the dorsal horns was nonessential, they were generally atrophic. These observations contrast sharply with the findings mentioned above (see "Random or Quasi-

Random Neural Networks") on the nonnatural motor outputs from similar deplanted spinal cord fragments in which either of the two above conditions was not essential.

These experiments show clearly that the motor programs for limb movement are built into the segmental apparatus of the limb-innervating parts of the cord and that they can produce rhythmic outputs even in the complete absence of neural connections with other parts of the CNS and also in the absence of efferent control. In contrast to the nonorganoid random deplants containing only 10 to 20 neurons (discussed earlier), which can produce only irregular bursts, real rhythmic output is produced by the organoid deplants that can be assumed to have retained much of the essential structure shown in Figure 15.

Perhaps it is not too daring to assume from this that a number of spinal gray matter modules stacked in correct order, and hence having a number of correctly interconnected interneurons, both excitatory and inhibitory, might be considered to be the very minimum of neural structure that can contain the program for coordinated limb movement.

In spite of the apparent usefulness of the modular concept in our spinal cord model, it is advisable to have a second look at the modular structure in order to appreciate how far the concept corresponds to straightforward structural reality as opposed to metaphorical paraphrasing. The reality, as mentioned, is the predominantly transversal orientation of the neuropil, both of the axonal and interneuronal dendritic arborizations. This would not mean, however, that the neuropil is, in fact, subdivided into flat transversal discs with empty septa between the neighboring discs. Such an impression might be gained from many longitudinally oriented Golgi sections, whereas the bundling of dorsal root (and perhaps also other) collaterals, emphasized by Scheibel and Scheibel (1969), might also contribute to this picture. This is probably due to shrinkage in the Golgi material that tends to break the neuropil into smaller compartments along interfaces of minor tissue resistance that obviously run in transversal planes in the spinal gray matter. The modular structure would be a reality in the literal sense only if a group of interneurons belong to one neuropil disc and not to another. No indication of this, however, is seen; in the longitudinal axis of the cord, there is a continuously shifting overlap between the flat dendritic trees of closely neighboring neurons. Hence, the modular concept should not be used here in the literal sense.

There are, nevertheless, many cases where a certain degree of "modularity" is introduced into neural tissue structure simply by the spatial independence (noninterpenetration) of nerve cells. As already mentioned, mutual invasion of each other's dendritic spaces is maximal in neurons of the isodendritic type of Ramón-Moliner and Nauta (1966) and tends to decrease towards the idiodendritic type. In most cases, though, this independence of dendritic space does not get very far, as there is still some sharing of the same tissue spaces by the dendrites of different cells. It is only in some of the precerebellar nuclei (see Figure 58) and (surprisingly) in certain cerebellar nuclei that a marked tendency during phylogenesis (and to some extent also during ontogenesis) to establish completely independent spaces for the arborization of the dendrites of individual cells is found. This trend reaches its peak in the inferior olive and the dentate nucleus of the cerebellum of primates, particularly of man (see Figure 125 of Eccles et al., 1967).

Cerebellar Modules

In the cerebellar cortex, the dense dendritic arborizations of the Purkinje cells are confined to flat boxes oriented in planes perpendicular to the longitudinal axes of the folia (Figure 16).* These spaces are not invaded by other nerve cells and dendrites, although they may show indentations in order to accommodate the cell bodies of basket or stellate cells and occasionally holes for the passage of capillaries (see Figure 10 of Ramón y Cajal, 1911). Apart from these, there is no interpenetration between the dendritic trees of neighboring Purkinje cells, on the contrary, there are narrow chasms between the large surfaces of the Purkinje cell "boxes" containing the dendritic trees of the local interneurons (basket, stellate, and Golgi cells). All kinds of axons (parallel fibers, climbing fibers, recurrent Purkinje axon collaterals), of course, penetrate through (or into) the dendritic spaces of the Purkinje cells. This aspect of cerebellar cortex structure has generally been known since the early classical Golgi studies. Interestingly, this separation does not seem to have any particular phylogeny; at least it does not seem as though the individualization of the dendritic trees emerged gradually in vertebrate phylogeny. The arrangement of elements and the regularity and economy in the use of tissue space are

*The reader unfamiliar with the cerebellar cortex will find the necessary background material in Chapter V.

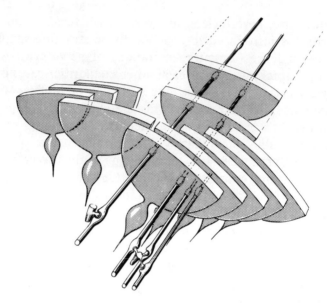

Figure 16. Spatial arrangement of the dendritic trees of Purkinje cells in the cerebellar cortex as deduced from the quantitative and stereological studies of Palkovits and his co-workers (1971a,b,c, 1972). Only about every fifth to sixth Purkinje cell stands in register in the longitudinal direction of the folium. The parallel fibers establish synaptic contacts (statistically) with about one in five dendritic arborizations of those Purkinje cells being crossed. [Szentágothai]

as ingenious (if not more so) in the lower vertebrates as in mammals. It would be ill-advised, though, to draw far-reaching general conclusions from the highly sophisticated structural development of the cerebellum in fishes, without taking into account the special modes of sensory reception in this class of vertebrates that are absent in the higher classes.

The cerebellar cortex is the most impressive example in the CNS of modular architecture appearing to be an essential feature. Although this interesting aspect has been discussed in some detail (see Chapter 9 in Eccles et al., 1967), more recent quantitative and stereological studies on the cerebellum of the cat (Palkovits et al., 1971a,b,c, 1972) have disclosed some interesting new aspects that are worth consideration. The Purkinje cells appear to be arranged in a staggered fashion (Figure 16); hence, about every fifth to sixth cell is standing in register with reference to the longitudinal axis of the folium (Palkovits et al., 1971a). Surprisingly, the parallel fibers, which are about 2 mm long on the average, establish synapses with about every fifth Purkinje cell whose dendritic trees they cross (Palkovits et al., 1971c). Since each

Purkinje dendritic tree is crossed by about 4×10^5 parallel fibers, the number of Purkinje cell-parallel fiber synapses was estimated to be 8×10^4 (with certain necessary corrections, 8.3×10^4; Palkovits et al., 1971c). By a completely independent and different approach, a later stereological study of the Purkinje cell spines showed 9×10^4 dendritic spines per Purkinje cell; this estimation is in remarkably fair agreement with that obtained by the earlier, more indirect approach (Palkovits et al., 1972).

These data make it possible to investigate further the mechanisms by which neuronal connectivity is engineered during development. Since parallel fibers (in rats and cats for example) grow largely during the first postnatal weeks, experiments were devised to study the development of these quantitative parameters by interfering with the normal function of the cerebellum (Pellionisz et al., 1974). The limbs of kittens were severely restrained (at 5 to 6 days of age) by placing them in casts made of a mixture of wax and paraffin, with heavy lead weights inserted into the soles. These casts virtually prohibited all limb movements (the hindlimbs more than the forelimbs) but did not interfere with their growth. These kittens were raised until the fifth week, at which time they showed a heavy ataxia when released from the casts, although their joints were not ankylotic and muscle atrophy was moderate. The cerebella showed major changes in the projection areas of the hindlimbs and minor ones only in the forelimb area. In comparison, similar control regions in normal littermates seemed to be unchanged. The main change was an obvious increase in the surface of the molecular layer section occupied by glia, and, interestingly, an apparent increase of section profiles of synaptic thickenings of parallel fibers as compared to the number of nonsynaptic (thin) profiles of parallel fibers. On the basis of the same stereological calculation that led to the conclusion that the average parallel fiber establishes synaptic contacts with every fifth Purkinje cell whose dendritic tree it crosses, it was concluded that, in the hindlimb projection area of the restricted kitten, the average parallel fiber contacts synaptically every third or second Purkinje cell crossed. A detailed stereological analysis of this material showed that the number of dendritic spines (9×10^4) per Purkinje cell remained unchanged. The ratio (1792:1) of parallel fibers (corresponding to granule cells) to Purkinje cell (Palkovits et al., 1972) was also unchanged. However, the length of the parallel fibers was reduced almost to half. In order to satisfy the unchanged number of available Purkinje dendritic spines, the number (density) of synaptic thickenings (contacts) per unit length of parallel fibers had to be increased nearly twofold.

This conclusion ought not to be generalized since the Purkinje cells appear to be exceptional in producing spines irrespective of any reduction in the number of parallel fibers (Hámori, 1973). Nevertheless, this case shows one possible strategy in the development of synaptic connectivity based on "supply and demand." The primary parameters, in this case, are apparently the numbers of Purkinje dendritic spines and the numbers and lengths of the parallel fibers. Normally, the total number of Purkinje dendritic spines can be satisfied by parallel fiber contacts if each parallel fiber establishes a synapse with every fifth Purkinje cell whose dendritic trees it penetrates. In the restrained kitten, the parallel fibers apparently do not grow to normal length; hence, the unchanged, total Purkinje cell spine number becomes much larger relative to total parallel fiber length available. Consequently, each parallel fiber has to establish contacts with every third or even every second Purkinje cell that it crosses. In terms of a genetically predetermined, developmental program, there would be no need for special instructions given to any parallel fiber with a Purkinje cell to contact, since the demand determined by the total number of Purkinje spines and the supply of so many granule cells (1792 per Purkinje cell) would automatically result in each 2-mm long parallel fiber contacting 1 in 5 (45 Purkinje cells) out of the 225 Purkinje cells encountered (Palkovits et al., 1971c, 1972). (This will also be discussed in Chapter V.)

The remarkable thing about the regular arrangement of the Purkinje cell modules is that *it makes the cerebellar cortex a quasi-crystalline structure in which connectivity is determined by the lattice constants.* A change in a single parameter (for example, the length of the parallel fibers) could change the whole connectivity in a systematic fashion. The change in connectivity could even be predicted by considering the neuronal growth processes that would occur during the period of the experiment. More important, the functional consequences of such connectivity changes could be studied in computer simulation models (see Chapter V) and the results could be compared with physiological studies in the same experimental situation. Although the situation is more obvious in the cerebellar cortex, owing to the regularity of the structure, it is not different in principle from that occurring in central neural tissue in general. The different kinds of central neural tissue are generally made up of a certain number of cell types, each essentially similar in size, shape, and arborization pattern. The repetition at determined distances of modular elements (even if the processes invade each other's spaces) necessarily leads to certain quasi-crystalline regularities; although these might not be obvious, they might be relevant for the internal connectivity of the network.

Modules of Specific Connectivity

A modular structure in a less literal (albeit no less realistic) sense can be introduced by certain specific actions, excitatory or inhibitory, of certain types of connections. The distribution of excitation and inhibition in modular spatial patterns, predetermined by the geometry of specific connections, was first envisaged in the cerebellar cortex (Szentágothai, 1963a, 1965). The idea of a longitudinally arranged population of Purkinje cells excited by a beam of simultaneously excited parallel fibers, flanked on both sides by "off beam" basket (and stellate) inhibition, became the basic concept underlying the operational features of the "neuron machine" of the cerebellar cortex (Eccles et al., 1967). The superposition of such functionally generated excitatory-inhibitory modules on an unfolded piece of cerebellar cortex (having a finite size of 2 X 3 cm) could be envisaged at that time as shown in Figure 123 by Eccles and his collaborators (1967). Although this diagram attempted to demonstrate the interactions of partially overlapping functional modules, it could not be further developed, owing to a lack of theoretical analysis at that time. As will be discussed in more detail in Chapter V on cerebellar functions, this aspect of network function is now within reach of both direct physiological experimentation and modeling by computer simulation.

The original simplistic concept of the functional excitation-inhibition module, however, must now be modified on the basis of the new quantitative observations. The two basic principles of arrangement and connectivity of structural elements, illustrated in Figure 16, require a radical reinterpretation of the modules in one crucial respect. The spread of excitation along a simultaneously excited beam of parallel fibers and the ensuing bilateral fringe of inhibition remain unchanged; however, the consequence of parallel fiber excitation on the activity of the Purkinje cells now appears in a completely different light. It is no longer reasonable to assume that two Purkinje cells closely adjacent in the longitudinal direction of the folium would be activated under identical circumstances. On the contrary, the out-of-register position of the dendritic trees of neighboring Purkinje cells and the statistically unlikely event that any parallel fiber has synapses with two immediately neighboring Purkinje cells in the longitudinal direction would lead us to predict that the receptive fields of closely neighboring Purkinje cells may be radically different. Interestingly, this prediction is clearly borne out by recent physiological observations (Eccles et al., 1971c; Llinás et al., 1971). This does not, of course, mean that the original modular concept is wrong or meaningless, but it does show that such all-over functional modules do not necessarily imply that all elements of the same kind within the module have the same functional roles. In fact, this restriction makes the modular concept even more attractive: in spite of a considerable sharing of a large part of the interneuronal machine (Golgi neuron mechanism of input control, basket-stellate lateral inhibition, etc.), there is ample room in the module to allow for subtleties in arrangement in close proximity to specifically different Purkinje cells. Since there is a definite somatotopic pattern in the projection from cerebellar cortex to cerebellar nuclei, the construction of neighborhood relations from Purkinje cells having specifically different receptive fields might be just the crucial principle on which cerebellar function is based. When considering the role of the cerebellum in the control of movement in Chapter V, these potentialities in its construction principle are worth serious consideration.

Such speculations on modules of spatial distribution of excitation and inhibition also offer tempting possibilities for the cerebral cortex. The first tentative neocortical models of this kind (Szentágothai, 1967a, 1969) were obviously still under the influence of (and isomorphic with) the cerebellar model, especially in regard to the distribution of inhibition. However, two basic features began to take shape: (1) the vertical intracortical spread of excitation seemed to be handled by Golgi type II interneurons, a possibility already envisaged earlier (Colonnier, 1966); and (2) the basket cells were the most likely candidates for inhibition, as supported by experimental anatomical (Szentágothai, 1962, 1965) and ultrastructural (Colonnier, 1968) observations. An interesting feature of the search for the neuronal basis of inhibition was the possibility of a "coarse grain" mosaic in the distribution of excitation and inhibition in the middle layers (laminas III to V) and a "fine grain" resolution in lamina II (Szentágothai, 1969). New observations on the distribution of basket cell axons in thin, vertically oriented slices (Marin-Padilla, 1970) led to an improved modular concept of the spatial distribution of inhibition (Szentágothai, 1970a, 1972a).

The resulting concept of a complex modular system of spatial excitatory and inhibitory actions is illustrated in Figure 17. This stereodiagram visualizes the translation of a focus of excitation, set up (in a primary sensory region) in a part of lamina IV by specific afferent activity, into a pattern of ascending and descending activity by Golgi type II interneurons within the two vertical cylindrical spaces in laminas III and VI. Parallel alignment between the ascending and descending Golgi cell axonal arborizations and (1) the apical dendrites of pyramidal cells as well as (2) the dendrites of fusiform cells in the deeper cortical layers would ensure relatively strong and specific excitatory actions on both pyramidal and fusiform cells within these cylindrical spaces. Large basket cells situated in the original focus of lamina IV (or in the secondary ascending and descending foci) would inhibit all pyramidal cells in vertically oriented parallel slices through laminas III to V, and thus contract (or otherwise shape) the tissue spaces within which excitation can develop under various circumstances. In lamina II a mosaic of smaller modular size can be demonstrated by the action of smaller, often octopus-shaped basket cells, the axons of which establish baskets around second layer, star-pyramid-shaped cell bodies in their neighborhood (Szentágothai, 1969, 1970b, 1973a). A newly found, specific Golgi type II cell (in lamina II and upper lamina III), labeled "chandelier cell," contacts the apical dendrites of pyramidal cells within a horizontally disc-shaped space that would correspond in size to the "bundle" of apical dendrites belonging to a pyramidal cell "cluster" as envisaged by Peters and Walsh (1972). Since the grape-like groups of terminal knobs are clearly arranged around the apical dendrites in a way that is suggestive of direct contacts with the surface proper of the dendritic shafts, and since, according to electron microscope observations, the synaptic contacts clustered around dendrite shafts in upper lamina III and in lamina II correspond to the AF (asymmetric membrane contact, flattened vesicle) type, it is not unreasonable to assume that the chandelier cells are another likely candidate for specific inhibitory neurons in the neocortex. In conformance with similar speculations made by Llinás and Hillman (1969) on the possible "functional amputation" of Purkinje cell dendrites by the action of stellate (and ascending basket) axonal contacts, one could visualize the action of the chandelier cells as a functional amputation of the upper part of the apical dendritic tree in

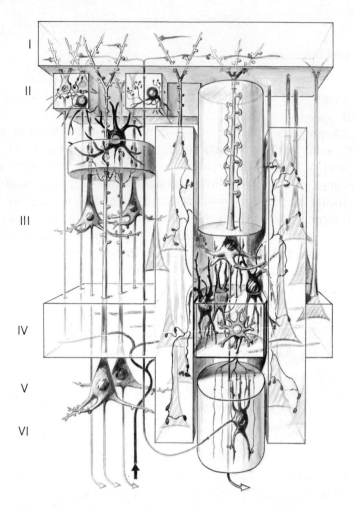

Figure 17. The basic neuron circuit of the neocortex with an attempt to delineate tissue spaces (modules) within which specific interactions between certain types of neurons can be expected. Assuming—by a suitable convergence of impulses arriving through specific afferents in lamina IV—an excitatory focus is created in the cylindric space (at right center) of this layer, this could be translated into a vertically ascending and/or descending volley through excitatory interneurons of the Golgi type II (stippled) in the two cylindric spaces in laminas II to III and V to VI. Some of these cells (the "cellules à double bouquet" of Ramón y Cajal) may have extremely powerful actions on a single (or very few) pyramidal neuron(s) by their multiple synapses around the apical dendrites ("cartridges" of Szentágothai, 1969). These first-order interneurons may be the simple cells of Hubel and Wiesel. Basket cells (solid) that would be stimulated by the primary (or possibly by the secondary) focus would be able to inhibit all pyramidal cells within parallel thin vertical slices of cortical tissue through laminas III, IV, and V, thus shaping (or partially cutting down) the primary and secondary foci of excitation. Smaller "octopus-shaped" basket cells (of small-range action) in lamina II could create a functional mosaic of smaller module size by inhibiting the small (star) pyramidal cells of this layer. A recently discovered (and presumably inhibitory) cell, at the border between laminas II and III, has been named "chandelier" cell on the basis of its peculiar axonal arborization. The terminal ramifications of the axon surround the dendritic shafts of pyramidal cells and establish synapses, containing ovoid vesicles, with the surface proper of the dendrites but not with the spines. Such cells, if indeed inhibitory, might functionally amputate the upper part of the dendritic tree in a cluster of pyramidal cells (in the flat cylinder-shaped box at upper left). [Developed from earlier diagrams of Szentágothai, 1967a, 1969, 1972a]

a cluster of pyramidal cells. (Note, however, the role played by functional amputation of Purkinje cells by climbing fibers in the Boylls model in Chapter V.)

Figure 17 cannot do justice to the many characteristic types of Golgi type II cells described by Ramón y Cajal (1899),* and several kinds are illustrated in a recent review by Szentágothai (1973a). The spatial actions and resulting modular subdivisions are much more diversified than can be envisioned for the time being. The possibility of histologically visualizing (by the injection of Procion yellow) cortical cells that have been previously identified with respect to their functional properties (receptive fields) will probably yield a wealth of new information that will support these concepts.

In contrast to the highly specific spatial distribution of (and hence connectivities established by) various types of interneurons, (1) the connectivity between the numerous axon collaterals of pyramidal cells *and* other pyramidal and nonpyramidal neurons, and (2) in lamina I the connectivity between the surface-parallel, terminal axon branches of association (corticocortical) or callosal afferents and the ascending axons of the cells in the deeper cortical layers *and* the branches of apical dendrites are arranged in such a diffuse manner that specific organization of spatial interactions cannot yet be imagined. Since there is no parallel alignment between zonal layer axons that cross the terminal branches of the apical dendrites, there is little, if any, probability that any given terminal axon has more than one or two synaptic contacts with the spines of any given pyramidal cell. (The overwhelming majority of synapses in lamina I are axon-spine synapses (Szentágothai, 1971).) In the case of the pyramidal cell-axon collaterals, a parallel alignment between their terminal branches and various types of dendrites would be conceivable. However, in chronically isolated cortical slabs, the easily recognizable pyramidal collaterals do not show any specific relation of that sort with dendrites. Their contacts appear to be established in a completely haphazard manner with whatever element (mainly spines) that happens to come into close proximity. Therefore, both synaptic systems should be envisaged as acting through some kind of "mass action." This conclusion may be questionable in lamina I, where systematic clustering of the pyramidal cells (in the sense shown by Peters and Walsh, 1972) might create some order in connectivity that is not recognizable by looking at the arrangement. A thorough stereological analysis might reveal here a definite orderliness as it did in the molecular layer of the cerebellar

---

*This almost forgotten aspect of neocortical structure has been reclaimed from oblivion by Colonnier (1966).

cortex. This is less likely in the case of the pyramidal axon collaterals, as clearly demonstrated in an illustration (see Figure 7 of Scheibel and Scheibel, 1970) of all collaterals of 3 neighboring well-stained pyramidal cells. This figure shows that the collaterals of only 3 cells, i.e., less than a quarter of the cell number in a cluster defined by Peters and Walsh (1972), produce a dense, but otherwise unstructured, "cloud" of terminal axon arborizations with a diameter of 3 mm throughout the whole depth of the cortex. A whole cluster would bring about a cloud of similar size but of much higher density. Hence, there may be much larger modules of mass action (corresponding to cylinders 3 mm in width) superimposed on the module system (shown in Figure 17), based on the spatial distribution of interneuron axons. Again, since such clouds of pyramidal cell collaterals issued from various clusters are shifted systematically according to the spacing of the clusters, interference patterns between the various arborizations might result in some large-scale order within the apparent randomness of the neuropil. The possible significant effect of interference and moiré patterns on the neuronal architecture has recently been considered, but only from the viewpoint of how apparent regularities of neuropil structure might come about (Ramón-Moliner, 1970; Szentágothai, 1972b). The possible functional consequences have not yet been considered.

The modular concept of the neocortex discussed here is at variance with another proposed by Globus and Scheibel (1967) (for a more recent discussion of their model, see Chow and Leiman, 1970, pp. 177-180). In considering the possible neural mechanisms of stereopsis, it will be advisable to keep in mind these two alternative hypotheses about the functional architecture of the neocortex.

Large-Scale Organoid Modules

A most impressive type of modular structure, the so-called *barrel* organization, was discovered by Woolsey and Van der Loos (1970) in the somatosensory cortex. Unlike any other structure discussed in this section, this organization is a clear subdivision in lamina IV of what is apparently a structural continuum of the cortex. These separate "cortical organs" function as receptors of information from corresponding, well-defined anatomical subdivisions of a complex sense organ on the periphery involving the whiskers. Figure 18 (Van der Loos and Woolsey, 1973) shows the cytoarchitectonic subdivision of lamina IV in the somatosensory cortex of mice, corresponding to the

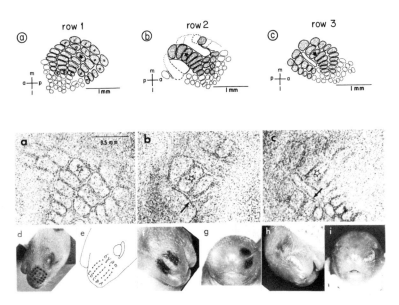

Figure 18. Cytoarchitectonic barrels in lamina IV of the somatosensory area (face region) of the young adult mouse. In row 1, diagram a shows a reconstruction from serial sections through the entire lamina IV of the barrel field; photomicrograph a shows tangential sections; figures d and e show placement, on the contralateral muzzle, of the corresponding large whiskers. Row 2 shows these arrangements after removal (and cauterization of the hair sinuses) of all but one row of the large whiskers. Row 3 shows the same after removal (and electrolysis of the hair sinuses) of one row of whiskers. Where vibrissae were injured at birth, corresponding barrels are absent in adulthood. In row 1, a code identifying the vibrissae barrels is indicated in diagram ⓐ and figures d and e. In row 2, in the barrelless region of diagram ⓑ, there are sheetlike assemblies of cells; where striking, they are indicated by solid lines; where less clear, by dashed lines; and where barely recognizable, by dotted lines. The stars in diagrams ⓐ, ⓑ, and ⓒ identify the starred barrels in photomicrographs a, b, and c. The arrows in photomicrographs b and c point to cell aggregates that occur where barrelless regions face intact barrels. a = anterior; l = lateral; m = medial; p = posterior. [Van der Loos and Woolsey, 1973]

large projection area of the whiskers. The cytoarchitectonic units are arranged in five rows (A to C) and correspond both in numbers and positions to the five rows of large whiskers on the contralateral side of the face (diagram ⓐ and figures d and e in Figure 18). The more numerous and less regularly placed small whiskers have corresponding smaller cytoarchitectonic units. The cytoarchitectonic units are called barrels because of their shape, this resemblance is most obvious if viewed in vertical sections of the cortex (Woolsey and Van der Loos, 1970). According to Golgi studies still in progress, this specific patterning in the Nissl picture is caused by the predominantly inward arrangement of the dendrites. The relation between the large whiskers and certain barrels was effectively demonstrated by more recent experiments in which the whiskers were destroyed at birth (all whiskers were destroyed except those in row C in figures b, f, and g in Figure 18; conversely, all whiskers were left intact except those in row C in figures c, h, and i in Figure 18); the corresponding barrels disappeared as a consequence of the subsequent transneuronal atrophy running through the whole ascending neuron chain. This is a unique example of the known trophic interdependence of even distant links in the neuron chain of the sensory pathways. But, as usual in such experiments, even this exceptional demonstration does not allow one to state specifically what was the consequence of functional deprivation and what was the consequence of disconnection with downstream links of the neuron network. What is so remarkable in this example is that separate units of a composite sense organ (a single large whisker is supplied by several hundred primary afferent fibers) have a well-isolated and structurally identifiable receptive organ in the sensory cortex, at least in lamina IV, which is the main receiving locus of specific sensory afferents. Therefore, this is a unique opportunity to study modular architecture on a large, quasi-organ scale, by a stepwise confrontation of structural and functional observations. It would be of particular interest to bridge the gap between the large-scale discontinuity in the cortical receiving areas of sense organs and the hidden discontinuities that are assumed in the receiving areas of the apparently more continuous receptive surfaces.

Layer-by-Layer Analysis

As mentioned above (and as set forth in Principles 4 and 5 of Chapter II), one of the most crucial features of neural organization is an apparently hierarchical superposition of layers in both the structural and functional senses. The hierarchical organization of neural centers is so obvious that it is almost trivial: the spinal cord, lower brainstem, upper brainstem, and cortex. Similarly, in the sensory pathways, there are the receptor level, several levels for local feature analysis, subcortical nuclear level, and several cortical levels. It is unnecessary to belabor this hierarchical lamination, but it is worth mentioning that there exists a rather strict topic relationship between any point in one level and a particular point in the next level, both in an upward and downward direction. If this topic relationship is not apparent, it is generally not because of its absence but rather because one of the somatotopically connected units may have its neurons distributed in layers of unusual geometry, as, for example, with slightly sloping vertical slices in Clarke's column (Szentágothai, 1961). Although it is by now generally understood that this topic relationship is rarely, if ever, a true neuron-to-neuron (i.e., point-to-point) connection in the literal sense, neuroscientists (as mentioned in Chapter II) still think mainly in terms of single-electrode results, i.e., as if two related phenomena occurring at corresponding points of two interrelated levels would give a full explanation of what occurs between the two. Everyone is aware, of course, that local neighborhood relations are important at each level; in the retina interactions are mediated by the horizontal cells at the level of the first synapse, by amacrine cells at the level of the second synapse, and by Golgi type II interneurons at the level of the lateral geniculate body (LGB). However, they are generally explained in terms of some mechanical type of interaction: adaptation, enhancement of contrast by lateral inhibition, or other improvement of signal-to-noise ratio. We must ask ourselves: Is that all there is to it? If we consider the observation on feature detectors in the retina by Lettvin and his co-workers (1959), then some kind of global analysis has to be expected. Even if such mechanisms do not occur in the retina of many higher vertebrates, similar ones invariably turn up at the next or further level. The search for organizational principles therefore, has to include the question of how the transmission and transformation of two-dimensional patterns from one layer to another might convey or extract meaningful information.

The cerebellar cortex offers a unique model for the study of this aspect of neural organization, simply by its exceptionally clear structural and functional lamination. Figure 19 shows this semidiagrammatically, with certain arbitrary changes in nonessential features; for example, the Purkinje (and basket) cells have been turned upside down in order to secure a consequent "bottom-up," input-output direction. In this form, the diagram seems almost trivial, however, it becomes useful for visualizing the transformation of spatial excitation (inhibition) patterns during transmission through the neuron network. It might be questioned whether one should compress elements such as the mossy rosettes, granule cells, etc., that are distributed in a relatively thick layer, into a two-dimensional layer. This depends, obviously, on the depth to which the conceptual (or computer) model of the network function requires such a consideration.

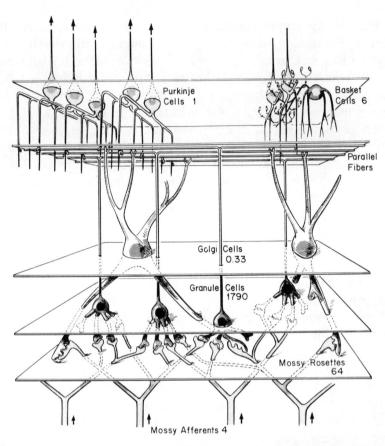

Figure 19. The neuron network of the cerebellar cortex schematically transformed into five two-dimensional matrices in which numerical, spatial, and connectivity relations of the several elements can be represented in a realistic manner. The only departures from reality are the compression of mossy rosettes, granule cells, and parallel fibers into a single layer, and the turning of the Purkinje and basket cells upside down to gain a consequently upward direction of impulse flow. The numbers indicated in the various layers are the numerical ratios of the respective elements to one Purkinje cell. [Szentágothai]

Eventually, a truly realistic model will have to consider the implications of the known fact that granule cells localized in the depth of the granule layer give rise to the parallel fibers in the deepest stratum of the molecular layer. Still to be carefully studied is whether the difference between superficial and deep parallel fibers in terms of the equivalent cylindrical dendrite model of Rall (1962, 1964) is sufficiently adequate to account for any major difference between their respective influence on the Purkinje cells. However, this is certainly not one of the major concerns of today's model builders. Thus, for the time being, the simplification introduced in Figure 19 appears to be permissible.

The layer-by-layer processing of impulse patterns can, indeed, be analyzed on the basis of Figure 19 by computer simulation (Pellionisz, 1970, 1972; Pellionisz and Szentágothai, 1973, 1974). The structural (i.e., connectivity, numeric, metric, and functional) parameters of the model network can be estimated from the microphysiological data available in the literature.

It would be naive, of course, to assume that direct information about the working of nerve nets could be gained from computer simulation models that do not make rich contact with structural and physiological data. However, contemporary literature abounds in fragmentary concepts or ideas, intuitively developed, on the possible modes of functioning of (1) specific neuron arrangements, e.g., the simple couplings of Lorente de Nó (1933) and whole circuits as shown in the drawings of Ramón y Cajal and other authors, and of (2) complete networks, e.g., the models of the cerebellar cortex of Szentágothai (1963a, 1965) and the models of the cerebral cortex of Globus and Scheibel (1967) and of Szentágothai (1967a, 1969, 1973a). Although such concepts are useful as guides for further experiments, computer simulation of the transformation of spatiotemporal patterns during their transmission from one neural layer to the next promises to be a powerful tool for prescreening and refining these concepts for use in biological experimentation. Many of the intuitive concepts on the operation of certain neuron couplings are easily disproved at the first step of simulation analysis. For example, the analysis of Golgi inhibition in the cerebellar cortex (Pellionisz and Szentágothai, 1973) clearly showed that direct stimulation of the lower dendrites of the Golgi cells by the mossy fibers is probably more important than the indirect stimulation of these cells via the upper dendrites by the parallel fibers. Moreover, this indirect stimulation is of little significance except as an additional means of filling in minor gaps in the spatiotemporal excitation pattern of the Golgi cells. More importantly, the possibility that parallel fibers are "preaddressed" to contact systematically only Purkinje cells that are in register (based on the observation that about every fifth Purkinje cell stands in register; see Figure 16 and Palkovits and co-workers, 1971a,c) was clearly refuted by a recent computer analysis (Pellionisz and Szentágothai, 1974). This new simulation model of the parallel fiber-Purkinje cell relay suggests that the spatial Purkinje cell activity pattern, resulting from neighboring foci of incoming mossy fiber activity, would show no meaningful differences whether (1) the parallel fiber contacts are systematically preaddressed to Purkinje cells standing in register or (2) the distribution of parallel fiber synapses is random, within the range given by the quantitative histological studies of Palkovits and his colleagues (1971c). Further predictions of this computer simulation will be discussed in Chapter V.

Similar arrangements of neuron networks in discrete layers occur in many parts of the nervous system. In vertebrates, the retina and the hippocampus are the most obvious examples of such arrangements. The behavioral significance of such layer-by-layer analysis of patterns can be observed in the retinotectal projection of lower vertebrates, which served as the evolutionary basis for the model of eye movements and visual perception discussed in Chapter II. In this system the additional advantage is that the transformation of sensory input into motor output is more immediate than anywhere else in the nervous system of higher animals.* Even better models for layer-by-layer arrangements of neural networks are available in the visual systems of invertebrates. Although their analysis has already yielded important insights into the principles of neural organization, their potentialities are far from exhausted. It is expected that they will yield the rich harvest only when the gap between structural-functional analysis and ethology is bridged, as some results along these lines already indicate (Land, 1974).

In most cases, however, the reduction of the neuron network to hierarchically ordered two-dimensional layers is not easily feasible nor would it offer any advantage for understanding the overall functions of the network. In the stacked chips model of the spinal cord network, for example, it would be meaningless to look for patterns successively transmitted from one chip to the other, because the chips are arranged and coupled in parallel relative to the main ascending and descending flows of information. In complex networks, as in the cerebral cortex, two strategies can be envisaged: (1) the global route, taken by Wilson and Cowan (see below), of considering the cortex as a quasi two-dimensional network by neglecting the vertical depth and interconnections and by looking for the horizontal interactions only, and (2) the detailed way, discussed above and in Figure 17, of breaking down the cortex into various types of modules that eventually might be reassembled into quasi two-dimensional layers.

*This system was discussed more fully at a recent NRP Work Session, "Sensorimotor Function of the Midbrain Tectum" (Ingle and Sprague, 1975).

Organization Principles of Afferent Systems

A particular advantage in studying the afferent systems is the opportunity they offer to search for the neural mechanisms by which features of biological relevance can be extracted from the immensely complex and constantly varying environment. Receptors, distributed all over the body and concentrated in strategic localizations corresponding to their specific transducing capacities, create a multiplex and rich mosaic of stimuli that are continuously transmitted to the centers over several millions of sensory channels. At the level of, or immediately beyond, the receptors there are several built-in mechanisms that improve the signal-to-noise ratios and/or ensure adaptation to excessive ranges of the physical parameters of the biologically significant stimuli. However, even at this level there begins the extraction of biologically meaningful messages from the total pattern of information flow. In some afferent systems, the feature-extracting process is confined to a single step. For example, in the frog retina, the convergence from the two-dimensional receptor matrix to the tectum is highly specific; these cells can be called "feature detectors." But to detect features of any degree of complexity, the feature-extracting process has to be accomplished in successive steps that are organized either in a hierarchical fashion or in parallel lines of processing. In the latter case, another sequence of higher order extraction might be envisaged as running across homologous points of the parallel chains, retrieving information not contained in any one of the channels but distributed over all of them. (This problem will be discussed again in Chapter IV.)

However meaningful this picture of the feature-extracting process might appear, it becomes inconclusive on further examination, since the nervous system has no "master file" or "final screen" in (or on) which the outer world is represented with any degree of isomorphism. So we soon end up with the basic mind-brain problem and that of conscious experience. However, this report (as was the Work Session) has to be confined to less ambitious aims. In our search for common organization principles in the afferent systems, we need to keep these thoughts in mind in order not to get lost in the often conflicting details of various possible strategies of information processing. Thus, in this section we begin first with an analysis of the similarity in the organization of linkages in the main sensory systems and then examine the detailed synaptic organization in the subcortical relay nuclei of these systems.

A Comparison of Neuronal and Synaptic Organizations in the Main Sensory Systems

Figure 20 gives a broad comparative view of neuronal arrangement in the subcortical parts of the main sensory systems. Details, especially of the spatial aspects of connectivity (divergence and convergence), are neglected in favor of principles of neuron coupling. Comparable levels of relay are presented as much as possible in the same horizontal plane; however, this is not always feasible owing to a lack of clear structural analogies among several systems. The diagrams for the olfactory system and the retinal parts of the visual system have

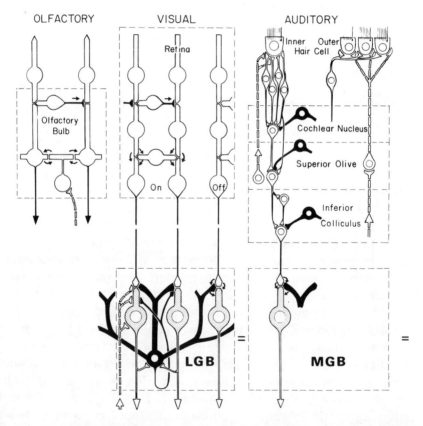

Figure 20. Grossly simplified comparative diagram of the elementary neuron couplings in the four main sensory pathways. Inhibitory interneurons are indicated by thick solid lines. Only general neuron couplings can be indicated in this diagram, and convergences and divergences are almost entirely neglected. Descending control is indicated by connections drawn in dashed outlines. In the primary afferent-dorsal column pathway (left diagram of the somatosensory

been adapted from Shepherd (1970). The diagram for the subgeniculate
portion of the acoustic pathway must be regarded as tentative, owing to
a lack of sufficient anatomical information. Sophisticated anatomical
information is available at the receptor and ganglionic levels, mainly
due to the studies of Spoendlin (1966), but our knowledge of the
acoustic system from the cochlear nucleus up to the inferior colliculus
is patchy. As one might expect, in any system in which frequency
discrimination is significant, introduction of "delay lines" into the
neuron net might be useful. Therefore, it is not astonishing to
encounter this mode of neuronal arrangement frequently in the
auditory pathway where a lower order afferent neuron divides and

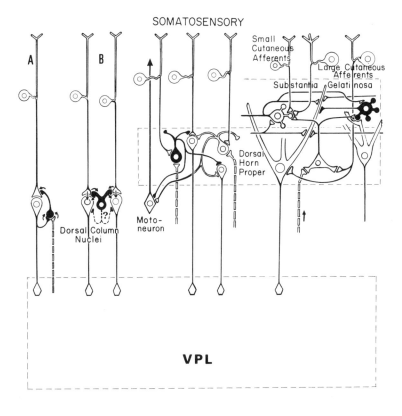

system), two possible interneuron couplings are indicated: A demonstrates the original concept
of an elementary recurrent feedback coupling, while B shows an arrangement using dendritic
synapses with triads. LGB = lateral geniculate body; MGB = medial geniculate body; VPL = ventroposterolateral nucleus. [Szentágothai; Shepherd, 1970]

reaches a two-step higher order neuron directly, and indirectly over another parallel channel through a neuron from the level in between. The shorter parallel neuron might be either excitatory or inhibitory; in both cases, such neuron coupling might be a useful frequency filter, as shown by the model experiments of Reiss (1964). The theoretical implications of these neuronal arrangements for the processing of auditory signals might be worth close scrutiny, although, as mentioned above in connection with another possible mode for frequency discrimination, the extremely narrow range within which such neuron coupling might be useful makes this possibility very remote.

The three parallel diagrams (Figure 20, right side) illustrating the somatosensory system are subdivided in order to account for (1) the dorsal column lemniscal system and (2) the anterolateral and spinocervical (dorsolateral) ascending systems. In these three systems, the connections in the upper brainstem are poorly understood: the anterolateral system has few direct terminations in the thalamus in subprimates, and very little is known about the supraspinal path. The involvement of the substantia gelatinosa is indicated only in the last diagram at the right of Figure 20; though it may play an important role in the anterolateral spinothalamic system, its involvement (in subprimates) is less obvious anatomically than in the spinocervical ascending system. One can feel surer of the lower part of the diagram, illustrating the neuron coupling in the subcortical relay nuclei, owing to many recent studies combining light (Golgi and degeneration) and electron microscope analyses. (This will be discussed in more detail below.)

The structural features illustrated in Figure 20 convey a convincing picture of the similarities in the basic neuronal mechanisms maintaining correct neighborhood relations of the essentially two-dimensional spatial patterns—joined by the changes in time as a third dimension—during their successive transmission to higher levels. However, they contain few, if any, useful cues for understanding how any global information can be extracted at these lower levels. Since we know, from the example of the retina of lower vertebrates, that such global information can be extracted, the search for such mechanisms has to continue. What has been left out of Figure 20 are the convergence and, in fact, all connections beyond the immediate neighborhood relations, which indicates how misleading such diagrams may be. There is enough detail in all of these diagrams to keep scores of physiological laboratories busy for years, exploring the fine neuronal mechanisms for sharpening contrasts or otherwise improving the signal-to-noise ratio, without giving the slightest structural hints for any more global kind of feature extraction. This is primarily due to the fact that the investigator of structure can better recognize and understand everything that is stereotypic and within close range than other investigators. Thus, conscious efforts are needed for a better understanding of the convergences and long-range cross-connections at the lower levels of sensory relay.

Recognition of frequency modulation at the single-neuron level in the cochlear nuclei (Erulkar et al., 1968) and movement detection at the retinal level in mammals (Barlow and Levick, 1965) are good examples of a transition from the mosaic type of receptive strategy to the global. For example, it is readily conceivable that certain patterns of frequency modulation are the crucial global signals that trigger or release complex behavioral patterns. Further investigation into the lower levels of the neural mechanisms of the various senses might reveal important shortcuts in the hierarchy of organized feature extraction. The question is whether such shortcuts will be exceptions to the general rule of hierarchical step-by-step analysis or, conversely, will eventually become an equivalent alternative strategy of feature detection.

Subcortical Relay Nuclei

A most remarkable degree of similarity prevails in the structural organization of the subcortical relay nuclei: the lateral geniculate nucleus in the visual, the medial geniculate nucleus in the auditory, and the thalamic ventroposterolateral (VPL) nucleus in the somatosensory systems. The similarity goes well beyond the principal analogy in neuron coupling that is indicated in Figure 20 (lower blocks).

The typical neuron coupling of the subcortical sensory relay nuclei is shown in Figure 21. The specific sensory afferent terminates (presynaptically) both on the dendrites of the thalamocortical relay cells and on dendrites (generally on specific dendritic appendages) of Golgi type II interneurons. The dendrites or dendritic appendages of the Golgi type II interneurons, however, are presynaptic in nature, i.e., they contain synaptic vesicles of the smaller ovoid or pleomorphic type and establish contacts of the usual presynaptic nature with dendrites (occasionally also with somata) of the relay cells. Understandably, these presynaptic dendritic profiles have been misinterpreted as axons in the early studies of the complex synaptic arrangements in the relay nuclei

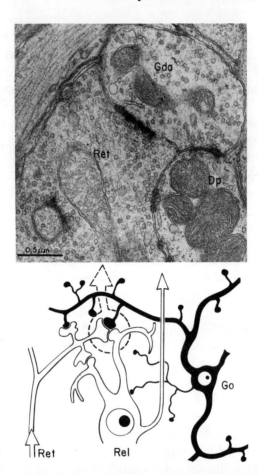

Figure 21. "Triadic" coupling of the subcortical sensory relay nuclei. Diagram at the bottom shows neuronal arrangement in the LGB, where a retinal (Ret) afferent terminal contacts both a dendritic protrusion of a geniculate cortical relay (Rel) neuron and the large dendritic appendage of a Golgi (Go) type II neuron. Electron micrograph at the top shows ultrastructural arrangement of the three neuronal constituents. Retinal afferent terminal is presynaptic (by contacts with round vesicles and asymmetric membrane attachments) to filamentous dendritic protrusions (Dp) of the relay cells and to the dendritic appendages (Gda) of Golgi type II neurons. The latter is again presynaptic (by contacts with flattened vesicles and asymmetric membranes) to the same relay cell dendritic protrusion. Scale, 0.5 μm. [Electron micrograph, Hámori, Pasik, and Pasik; diagram, Szentágothai]

(Colonnier and Guillery, 1964; Peters and Palay, 1966; Szentágothai et al., 1966; Szentágothai, 1963b, 1964a, 1970b). A full understanding of the dendritic nature of these presynaptic elements came from the studies of Morest (1971) on the medial geniculate body (MGB) and of Famiglietti and Peters (1972) on the LGB. It was finally recognized that what was earlier considered as an axoaxonic synapse is, in fact, axodendritic with a true axon as a presynaptic and a dendrite as a postsynaptic element (but the dendrite is presynaptic to another dendrite). A remarkable feature in these synaptic arrangements is the close association between three different kinds of synapses: (1) specific sensory afferent to relay cell dendrite, (2) specific sensory afferent to presynaptic Golgi cell dendrite, and (3) presynaptic Golgi cell dendrite (or dendritic appendage) to relay cell dendrite. The combination of these three contacts within close proximity had been recognized earlier, and speculations on the possible functional significance of these so-called "triadic" arrangements have been made (Szentágothai, 1970b). These speculations have now, of course, become obsolete through the recognition of the presynaptic nature of the postsynaptic dendrite in the synaptic glomeruli (or encapsulated synaptic zones) of the thalamic sensory relay nuclei (VPL, LGB, MGB); but we are still at a loss to explain the possible functional significance of this remarkable structural feature in the synaptic architecture of the relay nuclei.

There are, undoubtedly, certain similarities to the synaptic arrangements in the olfactory bulb and in the inner plexiform and ganglionic layers of the retina, but the functional explanation of these arrangements is also far from satisfactory. Also, it seems probable that similar arrangements exist in two other levels of the general somato-sensory pathways, where an abundance of apparently axoaxonic synapses has been found: the substantia gelatinosa and the dorsal column nuclei. So far, there is no direct evidence for this in the dorsal column nuclei, but studies in progress by Réthelyi* clearly show that most, if not all, of the so-called axoaxonic synapses in this region are, in fact, axodendritic synapses with presynaptic dendritic profiles. However, the occurrence of interneurons having presynaptic dendrites and being involved in such triadic synaptic arrangements, as shown in Figure 21, is not confined to the sensory pathways. Entirely similar interneurons and synaptic arrangements are found in other thalamic nuclei (ventrolateral, ventroanterior, lateroposterior, and pulvinar).†

The functional significance of the Golgi type II interneurons can be envisaged, for the time being, in three different ways: (1) effects localized within the neighborhood of a triad may influence transmission of activity from the sensory afferent axon to the relay cell dendrite; (2) activation of the interneuron axon may result in feedforward inhibition of the relay cells; and (3) activation of the interneuron dendritic tree may generate inhibition through the presynaptic dendritic sites.

*M. Réthelyi, personal communication.
†Studies on these nuclei are underway in various laboratories, and it is premature to include them in this discussion (e.g., see Hajdu et al., 1974).

By maintaining hundreds of presynaptic dendritic appendages, each interneuron is engaged in many triads (of the type shown in Figure 21) in its dendritic arborization territory and can, hence, influence the transmission from sensory afferents to relay cells in this whole region. In fact, there seems to be no synapse between the sensory afferents and the geniculocortical relay cells without the interference of at least one presynaptic Golgi dendritic profile. We do not know the role of this dendrite; but the original speculations of Pecci Saavedra and Vaccarezza (1968) and Szentágothai (1970b) on a presynaptic disinhibition role are probably not applicable, although they are not yet ruled out. In the discussion at the Work Session, Creutzfeldt suggested that such a triadic arrangement might serve as a device to transform the tonic discharge of the sensory afferent into a phasic discharge of the relay cell. This is brought about by the delayed inhibitory influence of the presynaptic dendritic profile upon the relay cell, triggered by the synapse from the sensory afferent to the presynaptic dendritic profile.

Another issue is whether these triads result in local activation of the interneuronal dendrite (as suggested by Famiglietti and Peters, 1972), or whether the entire interneuron is activated by the many synapses received from the sensory afferents. The two possibilities are by no means mutually exclusive. Since axons undeniably exist in most interneurons (Pasik et al., 1973), it is difficult to insist on a purely amacrine-type function for the interneurons.* However, since the interneurons have presynaptic sites both on their dendrites and on their axons, two possible mechanisms of overall interneuronal actions can be postulated: (1) a feedforward axonal inhibition and (2) a feedforward dendritic inhibition. In the first mechanism, activated interneurons may exert a feedforward inhibition through axons that terminate partly in the synaptic glomeruli but mostly on the cell bodies and even on initial axon segments of the relay cells. The interesting geometric consequences of the feedforward (or parallel) inhibition through the axons that are generally much shorter than the dendrites have already been considered by Szentágothai (1967b). Though feedforward inhibition is probably the predominant mode of interneuron action, it would not rule out the existence of a feedback type of inhibition, originally proposed by Andersen and Eccles (1962), which has a morphological basis in the initial axon collaterals of the thalamocortical relay cells

*This is controversial since Scheibel and Scheibel (1966) and Le Vay (1971) think that many interneurons are anaxonal.

(Tömböl, 1967). Note that the parallel inhibitory mechanism is not incompatible with mechanisms of cortical inhibition by the numerous cortical fibers descending to the sensory relay nuclei. Since cortical fibers terminate on both relay cells and interneurons, cortical facilitation as well as inhibition can be expected to exist.

Since the interneurons have many presynaptic sites (and contacts) distributed all over their dendritic trees, the second type of interneuronal inhibition, a feedforward dendritic inhibition, may also be proposed. If an interneuron is activated as a whole, it may liberate some inhibitory mediator from all of its presynaptic dendritic sites. Owing to the great length (200 μm and more) of the dendrites, this type of inhibition would have a considerably wider spatial influence than the axonal inhibition considered above. The geometric consequences of these types of possible actions have been recently considered by Hámori and his co-workers (1975).

It is obvious from these considerations that a large number of shaping mechanisms of the incoming sensory pattern by various types of inhibitory interactions could occur in this structural framework. Unfortunately, both neuron (relay and interneuron) types and the synaptic architecture appear to be rather stereotypic in all of the major subcortical sensory nuclei. Hence, the structure is not conducive to making deductions about specific mechanisms of more sophisticated or global feature-detection strategies. Although striking similarities in the elementary synaptic arrangements and in the two types of neurons involved exist, there are also considerable differences, especially between the modes of arborization of the specific sensory afferents and the arrangement in columns (LGB), laminas (MGB ventral division), and concentric spherical shells (VPL). These variations could introduce specific differences in the modes of convergence and divergence in the transmission from the specific sensory afferents to the cortical projection neurons. It is difficult to enter into even the most cursory discussion of this aspect. However, Figure 22 (assembled from the observations of Ramón y Cajal, 1911; Morest, 1965; Scheibel and Scheibel, 1966; Szentágothai, 1972b; Majorossy*) might convey an idea of the possible organization of the gross linkage in the main subcortical sensory relays.

*K. Majorossy, unpublished material.

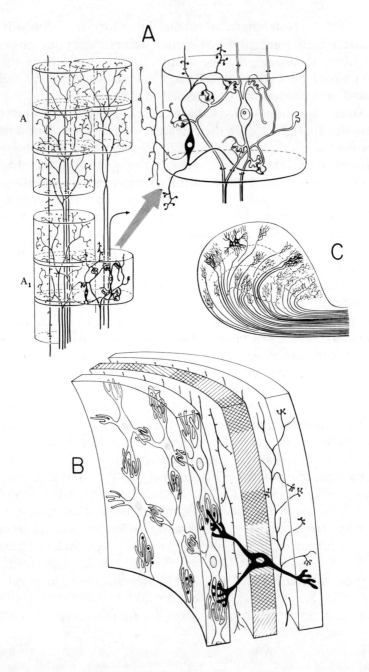

Figure 22. A comparison of the preterminal arborizations of specific sensory afferents that give some idea of the possibilities of convergence and divergence: in A, for the LGB; in B, for the MGB; and in C, for the VPL. [Szentágothai]

Organization Principles of
Internal Feedback Loops

As already mentioned, one of the fundamental organization principles of the system for the control of movement is the almost ubiquitous presence of internal feedback loops arranged in an interlocking multilevel fashion. This organization principle was discussed in an earlier *NRP Bulletin* by Evarts and his colleagues (1971, Chapter V), and this report reflects our present understanding of this important issue. In considering the overall role of feedback in the control of movement, that report distinguished three different types: (1) internal feedback, (2) response feedback (brought into action by receptors of the acting limb), and (3) "knowledge of results" (obvious as a phenomenon but not clearly separable, with respect to neural mechanisms involved, from internal feedback). The present discussion, since it is mainly concerned with general, structural organization principles, intends, instead, to consider neuronal feedback loop systems according to various degrees of complexity: (1) large-scale feedback pathways, (2) local (short-range) recurrent couplings, and (3) the possible structural basis of corollary discharge.

Organization of Large-Scale Feedback Pathways

The following three *large-scale loops* are generally included as part of the motor system:

(1) CORTEX → PONS → CEREBELLUM → VENTRAL THALAMUS (VL) → MOTOR CORTEX LOOP

(2) CORTEX → DORSAL COLUMN NUCLEI → MEDIAL LEMNISCUS → THALAMUS (VPL) → CORTEX LOOP

(3) THE "COMPARATOR LOOP":

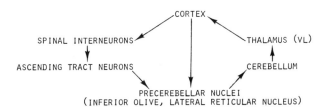

The general arrangement of these loops and their assumed functional significance as links conveying "motor command," "feedback," "command-monitoring," and "correction" signals have been summarized by Oscarsson (1973) in his excellent diagram (Figure 23).

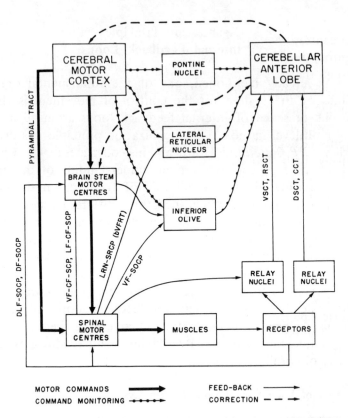

Figure 23. Some of the paths between the cerebral motor cortex, anterior lobe, and lower motor centers with an interpretation of the function of these paths. The anterior lobe is assumed to correct errors in motor activity elicited from the cerebral cortex and carried out by command signals through pyramidal and extrapyramidal paths. The command signals are assumed to be monitored by the anterior lobe through paths relayed in the inferior olive and pontine and reticular nuclei. The spinocerebellar paths are assumed to serve as feedback channels that monitor the activity in lower motor centers and the evolving movement. bVFRT = bilateral ventral flexor reflex tract; CCT = proprioceptive component of cuneocerebellar tract; DF-SOCP = dorsal spinoolivocerebellar path; DLF-SOCP = dorsolateral spinoolivocerebellar path; DSCT = proprioceptive component of dorsal spinocerebellar tract; LF-CF-SCP = lateral climbing fiber-spinocerebellar path; LRN-SRCP = spinoreticulocerebellar path relayed through lateral reticular nucleus; RSCT = rostral spinocerebellar tract; VF-CF-SCP = ventral climbing fiber-spinocerebellar path; VF-SOCP = ventral spinoolivocerebellar path; VSCT = ventral spinocerebellar tract. [Oscarsson, 1971]

The overall neuronal linkage of loops (1) and (2) needs little comment; however, it might be helpful to visualize the neuronal arrangement of the comparator loop in the spinal cord and precerebellar nuclei in some detail (Figure 24). The lower part of Figure 24, symbolizing the spinal cord, shows that the three different kinds of tract neurons (ventral spinocerebellar, spinoolivary, and spinoreticular) are essentially similar in organization in that they receive input from excitatory and inhibitory interneurons (which also have direct connections to motoneurons) that are, themselves, under strong descending cortical (and/or) brainstem control. The interneurons for the three different types of ascending tract neurons are not necessarily the same. However, since the sensory input to all these interneurons is from the flexor reflex afferents (FRA), these interneurons may be functionally similar, with relatively little modality specificity and with large receptive fields encompassing more than one limb (Oscarsson and Rosén, 1966). The direct cerebellar relay paths (dorsal spinocerebellar tract and cuneocerebellar tract) not taking part in the comparator feedback loop have a similar (excitatory and inhibitory) interneuronal organization, but they lack descending control and are directly and strongly driven by highly specific types of primary afferents (Oscarsson, 1973). (The functional significance of these large-scale feedback loops will be discussed in Chapter V; for details of their organization into distinct tracts, consult the review paper of Oscarsson, 1973.)

The comparator role of the system is twofold: (1) a comparison is made between descending commands and afferent inflow at the spinal level; (2) the output of the spinal comparator is transmitted to the medullary comparator centers, i.e., the precerebellar nuclei (inferior olive and lateral reticular nucleus), where a second confrontation occurs with direct descending commands from cortex and brainstem nuclei. To understand fully a comparison between descending cortical and ascending spinal patterns in terms of elementary neuronal and/or synaptic mechanisms, some information about the synaptic structure of these precerebellar nuclei is needed. The elegant Golgi studies of Scheibel and Scheibel (1955) may convey some insight into the spatial distribution of different afferent paths in the cat inferior olive. Unfortunately, the origins of these different afferents have not yet been identified. From cytoarchitectonics it appears that there are no local interneurons in the inferior olive; however, this does not eliminate the possibility of interneurons situated nearby. Indeed, physiological observations (Llinás, 1974) seem to suggest important mechanisms of local (perhaps recurrent) interactions. If inhibition is involved, one would have to consider the possibility that, instead of inhibition by interneurons, the cortical descending, the spinal ascending, or possibly unknown brainstem systems directly convey inhibition to the olivary neurons over long pathways. The local neuronal arrangement in, and the synaptology of, the lateral reticular nucleus are virtually unknown.

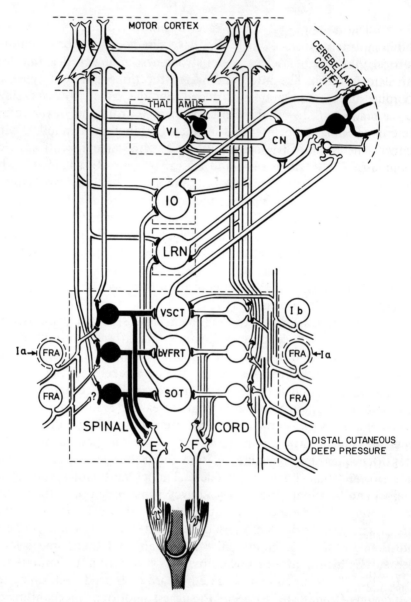

Figure 24. The main neuronal couplings in the "comparator loop" of the motor system. Diagram attempts to illustrate the convergence of descending cortical and primary afferent impulses on a set of spinal interneurons (the elements shaped like a Chianti bottle and arranged horizontally), usually lumped together under the term "spinal reflex center." They, in turn, project to the neurons of the main cerebellar ascending tracts (VSCT = ventral spinocerebellar tract; bVFRT = bilateral ventral flexor reflex tract; SOT = spinoolivary tract). The spinal interneurons are assumed to be either excitatory (open neurons) or inhibitory (solid neurons). However, they are not necessarily single neurons, ensuring a disynaptic connection from

The three large-scale feedback loops do not, of course, exhaust the complete list of such loops involved in motor control. At the Work Session, the participants did not seriously consider the large and intricate feedback loop systems involving the upper brainstem nuclei (corpus striatum and globus pallidus) and their projections to many lower brainstem nuclei. Although this omission can be justified by the time constraints of the Work Session and the space restrictions of this report, the reader should be aware of the limitations of such a summary.

Local Recurrent Couplings

The occurrence of recurrent local neuron couplings was first recognized by Ramón y Cajal (1911), and it might be appropriate to cite his phrasing of the general principle, explaining the recurrent couplings in his description of the cerebellar cortex: "Le second fait consiste en ce que le courant, qui passe par les cellules à cylindre-axe court, décrit fréquemment un trajet rétrograde et vient se déverser dans la voie sensitive ou sensorielle afférente qui lui a donné naissance." This principle was more explicitly stated by Lorente de Nó (1933), who, without our present knowledge of short (local) inhibitory interneurons, interpreted the recurrent neuron couplings as "self-reexciting chains" or "reverberating circuits." Another principle, that of "the multiplicity of connections" was simultaneously formulated by Lorente de Nó when he referred to the frequent mode of coupling in the relay nuclei in the CNS: the presynaptic fiber contacting the neuron (A) of the next link of a neuron chain gives a collateral to a short local interneuron (B), which in turn gives contacts to the same main relay neuron (A). Indeed,

---

primary afferents to ascending tract neurons and motoneurons; they may be chains of two or three neurons in which the final interneuron link may be inhibitory (since flexor reflex afferents (FRA) are the most general sources from the periphery). Two motoneurons, an extensor (E) and a flexor (F), are represented in the diagram. The connections are more complicated than can be indicated in such a summarizing diagram. Cases in which Ia muscle afferents have the same central connections as FRA are illustrated by a dashed circle, indicating that the Ia afferents would have larger spinal ganglion cells, corresponding to the larger diameter of their fibers. The other connections are the generally known pathways of the cerebellum (LRN = lateral reticular nucleus, IO = inferior olive; CN = cerebellar nuclei; VL = ventral lateral nucleus of the thalamus) with inhibitory interneurons coupled in parallel with the main synaptic fibers. The direct descending pathways are included, but many of them may be interrupted in the various brainstem nuclei (red nucleus, reticular formation, etc.). Aspects of laterality are entirely neglected. Ia = spindle primary afferents; Ib = Golgi tendon afferents. [Szentágothai]

we have here the two basic modes of local neuron couplings that can be recognized at almost all levels of neuron chains and in most of the more complex neuron networks.

The principle of recurrent neuron couplings reappeared in its inverse form when the existence of local inhibitory interneurons was discovered. Instead of "self-reexciting," the recurrent coupling became a circuit for "recurrent (or backward) inhibition" and the principle of multiplicity of connections became a circuit for "parallel (or forward) inhibition." The first mechanism of recurrent inhibition recognized was the recurrent loop of spinal motoneurons involving the Renshaw cells (Eccles et al., 1954a). Later, similar recurrent inhibitory mechanisms involving short-range neuronal loops were assumed in the sensory thalamic relay nuclei (Andersen and Eccles, 1962; Andersen et al., 1964). It became immediately apparent that both recurrent and parallel inhibitory couplings could serve through lateral inhibition as contrast-enhancing mechanisms, especially in the sensory system as well as in the Renshaw mechanism of the motoneurons (Brooks and Wilson, 1959).*

It was only recently that researchers in this field began to realize that what in the initial phase of the studies were viewed as relatively isolated elementary loops were, in fact, intimately interwoven with other mechanisms so that their isolation from the neural net in which they were embedded made them virtually meaningless. It has already been shown in the above discussion on subcortical relay nuclei that, although a local recurrent loop from the axon of the thalamo-cortical relay cell to the inhibitory interneuron may exist anatomically, it is embedded in an immensely complex network more suited for a forward inhibition (recurrent inhibition is principally generated by the corticothalamic descending system). That the Renshaw cell recurrent coupling is intimately interwoven with other inhibitory mechanisms of the spinal cord emerged first from the studies of Wilson and Burgess (1962) and Wilson and his co-workers (1964); however, the really revealing information came from the laboratory of A. Lundberg (Hultborn et al., 1971), showing that recurrent Renshaw inhibition is intimately coupled with the reciprocal inhibitory pathway from muscle spindles (Ia) to motoneurons. The fundamental significance of this coupling could be either (1) in "switching on and off" the inhibitory mechanism from extensors to flexors (and to some extent vice versa) through depression of the Renshaw cell activity in certain phases of

*See the analysis of the lateral eye of *Limulus* by Hartline and Ratliff (1957) and the review by Ratliff (1961).

stepping (Severin et al., 1968), or, (2) in securing the co-contraction of antagonist muscles by the Renshaw depression of the Ia reciprocal inhibitory pathway in certain supporting phases or in postural situations (Hultborn et al., 1971).

The Structural Basis of Corollary Discharge

Nothing discussed in this section could be interpreted as being a straightforward structural basis for the elusive corollary discharge. Although much of what is known about the segmental apparatus of the spinal cord could be viewed as conforming to the "reafference principle" of von Holst, there is no real need to try to "press" the marvelous refinement of a score of intricately interwoven neuronal linkages (see particularly Lundberg, 1970, 1971) into the procrustean bed of a single, too-general concept, however ingenious and fruitful it might appear. The many descending cortical connections (both excitatory and inhibitory) to the spinal internuncial (premotor and pre-descending tract) centers receive a more parsimonious explanation in Figure 24. The best fit with the general schemes in the literature on the flow diagrams explaining corollary discharge could be the connections from the motor cortex to the pontine nuclei, the lateral reticular nucleus, and the inferior olive (labeled command-monitoring pathways in Figure 23). Modification of neural computation, based on changes expected in sensory (i.e., external) or internal feedback as a result of a changed relationship between the body and the environment after execution of a motor command, is apparently a built-in part of the whole mechanism. After all, motor mechanisms from the lowest classical reflex type to the highest preprogrammed automatisms have developed during phylogenesis by continuous interaction with the environment. It may thus be a question of semantics whether the numerous and highly diverse neuron couplings subserving the very general purpose of monitoring efferent activity to modify afferent input ought to be labeled by a general term such as corollary discharge, which does not explain anything but does point out important differences between the control system view of the problem and its solution by the nervous system.

Tight Input-Output Couplings

In the classical neuroscience view, it was tacitly assumed that organization at the highest (cortical) levels is arranged essentially according to that at the lower levels: in the form of the "reflex arc" consisting of (1) an afferent (or ascending) limb, (2) a central apparatus primarily for funneling the afferent pattern into an efferent one, and (3) an efferent limb. This view is well illustrated by the diagrams of Ramón y Cajal (1911; see Figure 548). In considering, however, that the cortical regions receiving the main inputs from the principal sensory systems are not, in general, the same areas that are the chief sources of the corresponding motor output, the relation between the two cannot be that simple.

So-called "tight input-output couplings" were known earlier to exist in the sensorimotor cortex (see Evarts et al., 1971, pp. 51-56). Some recent information of crucial importance has been gained from the studies by Asanuma and Rosén (1972; Rosén and Asanuma, 1972), showing that adequate stimulation of skin receptors in the monkey's thumb was specifically funneled towards the groups of pyramidal cells in the motor cortex that give rise to the pyramidal tract fibers that project to the muscles of the thumb. These tight couplings are spatially arranged in a manner that would apparently be useful for the grasp reflex and the initial phase of the placing reactions. It had been assumed earlier that tight input-output couplings might be primarily involved in guiding or monitoring the movements in the tactile exploration of the environment (Whitsel et al., 1972). The corresponding functions in the visual system would be the steering of the eye to bring cuing arrays of features in the periphery into the fovea. But in reviewing the principal requirements of such a mechanism, it becomes obvious that a tight input-output coupling could never meet these requirements. Hence, one must be skeptical of the notion that such direct sensorimotor connections (even assuming an extremely sophisticated matching of columnarly arranged receptive field and motor cell assembly patterns) may fully account for the mechanisms monitoring movements for tactile, visual, or auditory exploration of the environment.

Therefore, it would be hazardous to generalize from the very elegant observations on tight coupling in the sensorimotor cortex to a general and simplified cortical reflex theory, even in the limited range of exploratory movements. Nevertheless, one could propose this as a marginal case within a wide spectrum of solutions, ranging from a simple reflex arc to complex systems as discussed in Chapter II and illustrated in Figure 3.

IV. STEREOPSIS

Stereopsis: The Perceptual Level

It requires time to pass from the appreciation of the *local* features (see the black and white regions of Figure 25) of a display to the perception of the global pattern (the Dalmatian dog) of which they are a part. This transition from disorder to order, in which interaction is required among the different regions, suggests that perceptual studies will find a powerful metaphor in the physicist's study of order-disorder transitions and cooperative phenomena.* In the case of ambiguous figures, the reversal may also be viewed as an order-disorder transition (to say the reversal is explained by such a transition would be an exaggeration). More interestingly, the perceptual transition exhibits *hysteresis:* once one has perceived an element in a scene, it is hard to change it. In the girl-crone picture (Figure 26), one locks into a state that can only be changed by consciously "relabeling" some local feature, but in the Necker cube (Figure 27) reversal is spontaneous.

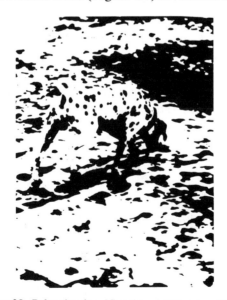

Figure 25. Dalmatian dog. [Carraher and Thurston, 1966]

*This metaphor was first introduced in Cragg's and Temperley's (1954) model for neuronal assemblies based on an analogy between the cerebral and the ferromagnetic structures.

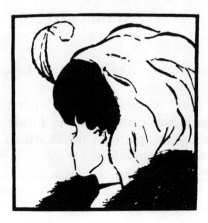

Figure 26. The girl and the crone. [E.G. Boring]

Global stereopsis exhibits order-disorder transitions that are very stable and can be destroyed only after the adaptation of local stereopsis units. Figure-ground reversal, according to Julesz, is not a cooperative phenomenon but just a simple shift in attention. For instance, when the vase-two faces figure (Figure 28) is portrayed by a random-dot stereogram, reversal of figure-ground cannot be voluntarily obtained. The closer area always becomes the figure, and, for figure-ground reversal, one has to reverse the disparities by exchanging the left and right images of the random-dot stereogram.

Julesz partly agrees with Pettigrew, who suggested that semantics may enter globally to aid region-by-region identification. When one tries to fuse a complex random-dot stereogram for the first time, it might take 1 or more minutes, since no familiarity cues exist. Of course, some semantics may be built into the stereopsis mechanism;

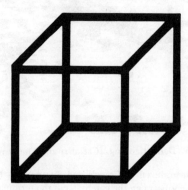

Figure 27. A classic Necker cube.

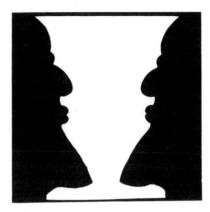

Figure 28. Figure-ground reversal. A vase or two faces. [Wyburn et al., 1964]

namely, any physical surface must be *dense*. Instead of searching for some "lace-like" surface (which can be obtained by small disparity shifts), the global stereopsis mechanism searches for a dense surface even if this requires large disparity shifts. Julesz (1971) finds that a random-dot stereogram portraying complex surfaces can be easily fused the second time (even after years of delay) because the subject remembers the range and direction (nasal or temporal) of the binocular disparity values. It is immaterial whether the object is a sphere, cone, or paraboloid, as long as it is portrayed at the same range and direction of binocular disparities. The reader can verify this by trying to fuse the random-dot stereogram of Figure 29 (Julesz, 1971). In spite of the fact that the reader is instructed to find a hyperbolic paraboloid (a saddle surface) and a torus above it, fusion is not speeded up.

Julesz's (1971) work on "cyclopean perception" shows that fusion of the two retinal images must precede pattern recognition. Many acts of perception cannot be mediated by the two eyes separately but require the fusion of their two patterns—as in the "eye of the cyclops." Viewed purely in terms of local features, the fusing of the images involves many ambiguities (Figure 30). Julesz (1971, pp. 187-198) has, in fact, developed techniques for generating pairs of random-dot patterns that yield ambiguous stereograms even at the level of *surfaces*, i.e., the two patterns are compatible with two different stippled objects. Yet humans can separate one from the other. However, the process (with or without ambiguity) takes time until the object suddenly stands out. One seems to go from overmatching of local features to just those appropriate to the perceived three-

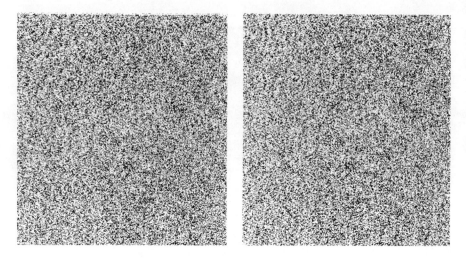

Figure 29. Random-dot stereogram of a complex surface. [Julesz, 1971]

dimensional object. It should be stressed, however, that, if the object is complex, the process can take 1 min, with more and more surfaces becoming defined as time progresses, i.e., the object need not be recognized in a single phase transition.

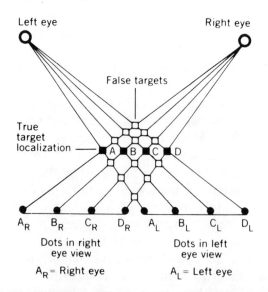

Figure 30. Ambiguities in global stereopsis arise when four targets (having the same ordinates) cast their projections on the left and right retinas. If these targets are similar, i.e., have the same brightness, color, shape, and orientation, it is ambiguous which projected target in one view belongs to which projection in the other eye's view. In the case of four targets, sixteen localizations are possible, of which only four are correct and twelve are "phantom" targets. With increased number of targets, the probability of false localization quickly becomes unity. [Julesz, 1968]

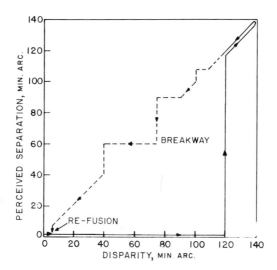

Figure 31. Hysteresis for a random-dot stereogram. [Fender and Julesz, 1967]

A classic experiment in fusion showed that a pair of dots—one projected into each eye—must lie within a 6 min arc (a region known as Panum's area) in order to be perceived as a single point. Fender and Julesz (1967), repeating this same experiment, demonstrated that, once fusion is obtained, it perseveres until the dots are pulled to about 120 min apart—a clear case of hysteresis. They also found the same effect with random-dot stereograms (Figure 31). The hysteresis effect is much smaller with a vertical line, demonstrating that global stereopsis (see Figure 32) is a cooperative phenomenon that depends on the complexities (number of elements) of the stereograms.

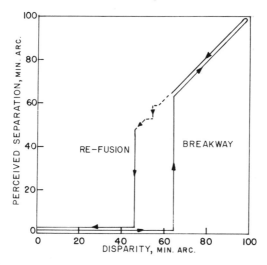

Figure 32. Hysteresis for a vertical line target. [Fender and Julesz, 1967]

The Cortical Neurophysiology of Stereopsis

Retinal ganglion cells show some resemblance to corresponding subsystems in somatosensory afferents, e.g., some are tonic, others, movement-sensitive, etc. Two main classes of retinal ganglion cells exist: the X class, which has large dendritic fields, and the Y class, which has small dendritic fields (Brown and Major, 1966). Stone and Hoffmann (1972) found that X and Y cells project mainly to cortical simple and complex cells, respectively, whereas W cells (a newly described class of very small cells that are direction-sensitive and whose axons have very low conduction velocities) project only to tectal structures (together with some Y cells).

The projections from the retina to the lateral geniculate nucleus (LGN) appear to be primarily excitatory; but the interactions between LGN cells appear to be exclusively inhibitory (Fuster et al., 1965; Creutzfeldt, 1968; Singer and Creutzfeldt, 1970; Singer et al., 1972). The LGN cells are driven by a very small number of afferent fibers. In fact, many are driven by only one afferent fiber (Creutzfeldt, 1968; Cleland et al., 1971; Levick et al., 1972), though some may be driven by a very small number of afferent fibers. In fact, inhibitory input, which involves triads within the LGN, is mixed. On-center and off-center excited cells are inhibited by both on-center as well as off-center cells whose receptive fields are identical with or surround that of the inhibited cell. Owing to this arrangement, not only lateral inhibition in the spatial domain but also successive inhibition in the temporal domain are found in the LGN (Singer et al., 1972). In many respects the response of these cells can be described as a differentiation of the retinal input, and their transfer properties can be modulated by arousal, etc. The columns in the LGN are a result of the ordered projection of the retina to the LGN (Sanderson, 1971). However, there is a scatter of 1° to 3° in the afferent input to a column. (There are 5 to 10 cells per layer in a microelectrode penetration; multiplication by 10 gives the average number of cells in a column.)

In the cortex, superimposed on the retinotopic map is a map of contour orientation, where the orientation changes systematically and occasionally reveals discontinuities. There may be variations in optimal orientation within a single column, but they are at the noise level in magnitude compared with the jumps in optimal orientation between columns. But it should be realized that orientation columns are not circular in cross section; their shape is elongate and more "sausage-like"

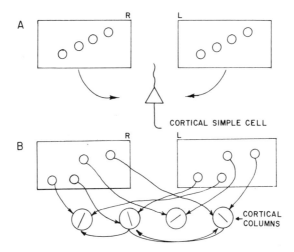

Figure 33. A. The classic model: receptive field location of right- and left-eye innervated LGN cells converging on one cortical "simple" cell. B. The Creutzfeldt model: receptive field location of LGN cells, each of which excites only one individual cortical cell. The cortical network properties determine the orientation and direction sensitivity of each cortical cell. See Figure 34 for further details. [Arbib and Szentágothai]

(Hubel and Wiesel, 1963).* The distance between the jumps in orientation, 200 to 500 μ, corresponds to the diameter estimated for the columns. Hubel and Wiesel suggest that orientation selectivity is the result of appropriate connectivity from the LGN, and that sharpness of selectivity depends on appropriate inhibition from the LGN (Figure 33A).

Benevento and his co-workers (1972), as well as Blakemore and Tobin (1972) and Blakemore and his collaborators (1970), suggest that input from the LGN can determine only the gross orientation to which the cell responds. In fact, at the Work Session Creutzfeldt presented material showing that the shapes of excitatory fields of cortical cells are usually not elongate and are generally not different from geniculate fields. He proposed that an asymmetrical arrangement of lateral inhibition in the cortex is responsible for the orientation and direction sensitivity of cortical cells. There was some disagreement among the participants about this, and Blakemore suggested that orientation-sensitive inhibition only sharpens the response of a cell along the dimension of orientation.

Creutzfeldt presented an intra- and extracellular analysis of cortical neuronal responses in such a way that individual cortical

*K. Albus, manuscript in preparation.

neurons could be excited by only one afferent LGN fiber from each eye, and that all other functional properties of cortical cells could be due only to inhibitory and, maybe, excitatory network properties of the cortex itself (Figure 33B). He confirmed, and elaborated on, the earlier observation of Hubel and Wiesel (1963) that the retinotopic map becomes "fuzzy" at the cortical level. In fact, the excitatory fields of cells in one cortical column are not identical, which suggests that each cortical cell has its "private" and discrete excitatory input line. This observation corresponds well with the random binocular convergence on individual cortical cells. Creutzfeldt also added that a binocular cortical map based on the classic model of Figure 33A would involve too much connection specificity.

The fact that intracortical inhibition has essentially the same properties as intracortical excitation, i.e., orientation-direction-movement sensitivity, does not exclude, of course, spatial aspects of intracortical inhibition as demonstrated by several investigators. Even if the retinotopic representation in area 17 is fuzzy, a retinotopic gradient is clearly recognized. This may be schematically demonstrated, as in Figure 34, where it is assumed that cortical cells are most probably excited from their corresponding retinal point, but that other points may also make tight excitatory contacts. If an orientation sensitivity map is drawn on such a fuzzy space map, and if it is assumed that, irrespective of columnar borders, cells within a certain diameter will inhibit each other, the two aspects of cortical inhibition—space and stimulus specificity—can be easily deduced.

Creutzfeldt's presentation elicited a variety of comments from the participants. MacKay cautioned that, in talking of fuzzy or random connections or orientations, one must not confuse undetectability of order with absence of order. He added that, in many electronic circuits, connectivity is everything and physical layout of the wiring is largely irrelevant. But in the CNS this is not so; thus, one must examine ways in which "proximity" may be important in organizing processing. Moreover, the forms of representation of information are such that being "neighbors in space" results in useful interaction between neurons. For example, proximity in space is useful in the extraction of spatial features such as lines and in the computation of movements related to orientation, e.g., where to move the eyes. It should be noted, however, that owing to the overlapping of dendritic and axonal fields, proximity may not be the appropriate word to use; two cells with perikarya that are far from each other may have processes that are close or even touching (Ramón-Moliner and Nauta, 1966).

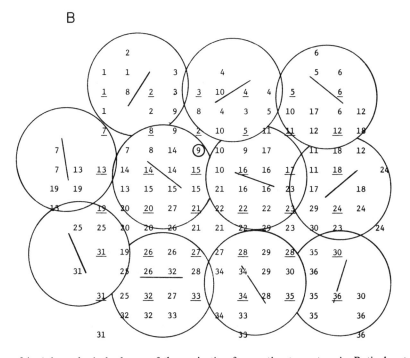

Figure 34. A hypothetical scheme of the projection from retina to cortex. A. Retinal matrix. Points on the retina are represented by numbers and may correspond to the receptive field centers of individual retinal ganglion cells. B. A hypothetical cortical spatial (numbers) and orientation (circles) matrix. It is assumed that each retinal point is projected to four cortical points. The retinal numbers were allocated to cortical points according to a weighted random matrix. The faithful retinotopic map is preserved with a probability of 4/7 (underlined numbers). Outside these points each fiber is connected to the next points with a probability of 2/7, and to the next further points with a probability of 1/7. If, during the sequential allocation of retinal numbers to cortical points, a point was already occupied, another free point was selected from the probability matrix. Thus, the map shows a certain fuzziness but a well-preserved "retinotopic gradient." A circle is drawn around groups of cortical points that have functional properties in common, (i.e., orientation sensitivity, as indicated by the lines). Each point may represent one cortical neuron that receives its primary excitatory input from the retinal point (or ganglion cell) indicated by the number. [O.D. Creutzfeldt, U. Kuhnt, and L.A. Benevento]

Blakemore suggested that maps other than retinotopic and orientation maps may exist, e.g., discontinuous maps of disparity and even, perhaps, of spatial frequency. These cortical cells, detecting various features such as orientation disparity, etc., may all benefit from a common process of spatial lateral inhibition.

At this point, the crucial question about the structural organization of the visual cortex to be asked of the anatomist is: "How much convergence, i.e., how many specific sensory afferents, is needed in order to ensure the trigger features experienced in the simple cells of primary sensory cortices?" Lacking any numerical information on the input-output ratios in the primary sensory cortices, it would be extremely hazardous to make guesses. However, from the strict somatotopic organization of the geniculostriate projection and the sparse arborizations (one or two arborizations) of the specific afferents before entering the cortex (Figure 14 in Szentágothai, 1973a), one might venture to conclude that the convergence cannot be in the order of hundreds. There is certainly nothing in the histology of the terminal arborizations (see Figures 21 and 22 in Ramón y Cajal, 1899; numerous figures in Lorente de Nó, 1922; Figure 14 in Szentágothai, 1973a) that suggests the massive termination of any given specific afferent on any cortical cell, and, hence, would lead to the conclusion of a very low convergence (on the order of two to three). However, the histological picture (even including the sparse degeneration seen under the electron microscope) may be misleading. A tentative guess (with many reservations added) might lead us to the assumption of a convergence of somewhere around ten for the average simple cell. However, this figure is still one order of magnitude larger than that postulated by Creutzfeldt; thus, further research is necessary. Inhibitory interactions at the level of the second intracortical synapse, as shown in Figure 17 in Chapter III and also suggested on the basis of physiological observations (Benevento et al., 1972; Blakemore and Tobin, 1972), might add additional refinements (e.g., direction and movement sensitivity) and might further reduce the numerical convergence requirements to the level proposed by Creutzfeldt.

Disparity-Tuned Neurons

Findings on disparity-tuned neurons reveal the following: paradoxically, the more binocular the mammal, the clearer the segregation into discrete layers of the input from the two eyes to the lateral geniculate, though there does exist inhibitory interaction between the two types of layers. Only at the cortical level is there a convergence of excitatory input from both eyes. In the 1950's Jung (see his 1961 review article) described some aspects of binocularity; later more detail was recorded by Hubel and Wiesel (1962), who noted that the cells might be biased to respond better to input from one eye than from the other. Cells in area centralis have very fine trigger features and require a specific orientation, stimulus width, etc., for maximal response. (Note that there is much "silence" in primary sensory cortices and many cells can be missed if spontaneous activity is expected. It is thus necessary to stimulate diversely as the electrode is advanced.) The optimal stimulus for a given cell is almost the same for each eye. This suggests that local features in the eyes can be easily matched; in natural scenes it is unlikely that two similar trigger features will be nearby, and so a cortical cell's response is most likely to be to the two retinal projections of the same spatial feature. This is not true, however, for "unnatural" stimuli such as random-dot stereograms (see the model discussed below) or for gratings.

But how does such a cell respond to disparity—the key local sign for stereopsis? The answer is that cells appear tuned for disparity. They respond best to a trigger feature when it is presented to both retinas with a certain disparity; as the disparity changes from the optimal value, the response decreases. (What connectivity would yield this effect?) The tuning for disparity in simple cells is very sharp ($\pm\frac{1}{2}°$). Moving up the "hierarchy," a complex cell generalizes optimal orientation located in a region extending over $6°$, but activity falls off for disparities of $\pm1\frac{1}{2}°$, though the falloff may be much broader for some "untuned" complex cells. Complex cells are now identified with pyramidal cells (Van Essen and Kelly, 1973). However, there are many cells that respond over a wide range of orientation and disparity. These may be basket cells playing a role analogous to that of Creutzfeldt's inhibitory interneurons (working in "disparity space") and this might explain why one complex cell can belong to three different columns.

Disparity introduced by a misalignment of the two eyes must be ignored for the purpose of depth perception; yet this disparity may drive disjunctive eye movements. Pettigrew's model (Figure 35) shows how these two functions may be obtained. The system controls disjunctive eye movements by preventing binocular interaction through interlaminar inhibition until disjunctive eye movements bring the retinal images into register. Such a system can be progressively refined

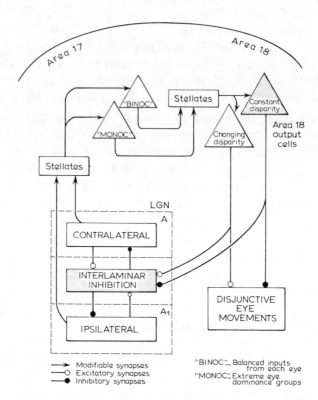

Figure 35. A model to show how highly specific binocular connections could be set up in the developing visual system by experience. The essential feature is that synchronous binocular activity of the cortical input be controlled by inhibition at the LGN concurrently with the relative alignment of the two eyes. Ocular misalignments (*disjunctive eye movements*) produce changes of retinal disparity as do objects in real depth, so binocular information transfer is prevented except when the eyes have the least tendency to swing apart. LGN *interlaminar inhibition,* which limits binocular synchrony, is greatest when the eyes are moving out of alignment and is decreased by the effects of the *constant disparity* neurons that are active when the eyes tend to be aligned. The cortical neurons of areas 17 and 18 have modifiable connections that become increasingly precise as the eye-movement conditions under which synchronous binocular activity to them become better defined, develop. In conditions of monocular stimulation (like eye occlusion) interlaminar inhibition is very strong because *constant disparity* neurons are not active, and developing cortical connections would rapidly begin to favor the stimulated eye. [Pettigrew, 1972a]

with experience. How do we relate this to columnar structure, cumulative buildup of patterns, and cooperative phenomena? Suppression via interlaminar inhibition may prevent the perception of "ghosts" in random-dot patterns. Further suppression of areas of poor correspondence in the disparity of retinal images may occur through lateral inhibition in the disparity domain, as shown in the Dev model below.

Positive feedback may contribute to an increase of activity in regions of good correspondence. Thus, a rough hierarchy of stereopsis mechanisms is obtained from local ones, such as activation of a disparity-sensitive cell, to global ones, such as detection of regions of constant disparity; but semantic information may be still needed. It may be that increased speed in the recognition of random-dot stereograms may involve "semantic feedback" (cf. the discussion on "nested analysis" below). However, as mentioned above, Julesz finds that, when there are many depth planes, knowing which binocular disparities portrayed the object helps to fuse it. This does not help with amorphous shapes, and for simple objects no semantic feedback is necessary.

Blakemore restricted his discussion and conclusions to the cat visual system, in which the visual information is filtered through line detectors. He suggested that there may be two hierarchies in the line-by-line analysis of disparity in the cat. The first hierarchy is as follows:

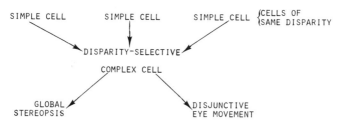

The machinery for this kind of organization can exist in the physiologically defined "constant depth" columns, in which the cells detect lines of the same orientation and the same disparity. It can be said that any such column "views" a certain "surface" in space. Moreover, these columns may be the basis for arriving at global stereopsis if there is inhibition between columns detecting different surfaces in space; the column that is maximally activated will inhibit other inappropriately activated constant depth columns. (See the discussion of the Dev model below.)

Creutzfeldt pointed out, however, that the simple-complex-hypercomplex, etc., hierarchy of visual cortical neurons is only a hypothesis, and that direct experimental proof of such an organization is yet lacking. Hubel and Wiesel (1962, 1965, 1968) have suggested such a hierarchical organization as a plausible explanation for the observation of neurons with trigger features of various complexity; but recent findings from several laboratories (Creutzfeldt et al., 1971;

Blakemore and Tobin, 1972) indicate that this purely hypothetical
model has to be at least revised if not fully changed. Nonetheless,
Blakemore suggested a second such hierarchy:

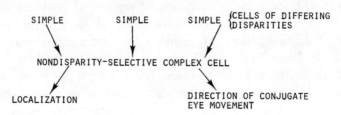

The reason for proposing the second hierarchy is that experimental results show that there are many columns with superimposed
receptor fields for projections from one eye but with a large spread of
horizontal disparities. If these cells converge on one complex cell, the
cell will be specific for positions in the same direction but at various
depths along that direction. Such information could, in turn, direct
conjugate eye movements (Blakemore, 1970b).

Thus, there may be two hierarchies that are disparity-selective
up to the simple cell level. However, there may be other parallel
hierarchies involved in stereopsis that are based on other types of
feature detectors. Such detectors could be specific for interocular
differences in width, orientation, length, direction of movement, or
velocity, as well as position (Blakemore et al., 1972).

In this context, two aspects should be kept in mind. One is a
suggestion made by Burns (1968) that the function of the disparity-
sensitive cells of area 17 is to search for a convergence position of the
eyes ideal for binocular fusion of an image at a certain distance. The
best convergence position is reached when a maximum of cortical cells
discharges maximally while looking at a certain object. The second
aspect is that, in primates, binocular disparity detectors are abundant in
the peristriate cortex (Hubel and Wiesel, 1970), whereas in cats this
seems to be a specialty of area 17 neurons. This further demonstrates
the aspects of parallel processing discussed in Chapter III.

Disparity-selective cells discussed so far are specific with respect
to position and measure differences of position in the corresponding
images. However, Pettigrew (1973) has data showing the existence of
cells that are direction-specific when the images from the two eyes
move in opposite directions. This could signal a stimulus moving
directly to or from the animal and, perhaps, provide a pathway parallel
to the position pathway for three-dimensional organization. Similarly,

Blakemore and his colleagues (1970) have found cells with different (up to 15°!) preferred orientations on the two retinas, presumably corresponding to a tilt of a contour towards or away from the observer. Their conclusion is that the cat may analyze various aspects of visual stimuli by parallel pathways, such as the above, for approach-retreat and tilting, and that every cell that is selective to one of the dicussed features may carry information about the third dimension. Is there a further hierarchical level at which the information from these various pathways is pooled? Note that such a level could well comprise an "action-oriented array" rather than a layer of "grandmother" cells.

Development of Visual Cortex Circuitry

Based on experiments with kittens, Pettigrew (1972a, 1974a,b) suggests that there is a progressive tuning of disparity selectivity during the third and fourth weeks of development. Whereas at 16 days the cells are very broadly tuned, by 30 days tuning is almost as sharp as that in an adult. Furthermore, normal development of inhibition of nonoptimal disparity requires visual experience.

Creutzfeldt cited a model developed by Malsburg (1973) in which the development of orientation-tuned cells is simulated by a learning network of cortical elements. The cortical elements are connected to each other by excitatory lines over small distances and by inhibitory lines over wider distances. At the beginning, the cortical network is connected to a retinal plane with random connections between retinal and neural cortical cells. Excitations of rows of retinal cells representing different orientations are simulated. Connections are made tighter according to Hebb's (1949) learning principle, i.e., a synapse is strengthened each time an afferent discharge occurs with a supra-threshold response of its cortical cell (synapses on a cell are renormalized after each adjustment). After 20 to 50 learning steps, most cortical cells are tuned to a certain orientation, and it turns out that cells lying close to each other are sensitive to identical or similar orientations, whereas further separated cortical cells are tuned to different orientations. After about 100 learning steps, a regular columnar matrix results, as in the real cortex.

Spinelli and Hirsch (1971; Hirsch and Spinelli, 1971) have shown that, if kittens are shown vertical lines through one eye and horizontal lines through the other as the only visual stimuli during development, a remarkable thing happens. On recording from single

cells in their visual cortex, one finds only two types of cells: (1) a
diffuse type, i.e., cells that have very weak responses to visual stimuli,
are nonselective for bars and/or edges of any orientation, and have no
clear receptive field when mapped by Spinelli's computer method, and
(2) cells with elongate receptive fields that are either vertical or
horizontal. If vertical, they can be mapped only through the eye that
has seen horizontals. In some of the experiments, it was observed that
some receptive fields looked remarkably like the recognizable images of
the bars seen by a kitten in its infancy!

Blakemore and Cooper (1970) exposed two kittens to cylinders
painted with vertical or horizontal stripes. When tested for orientation
sensitivity, cells in the visual cortex of the kitten that had been in the
horizontal cylinder responded best to lines that approached the
horizontal; cells in the cortex of the kitten in the vertical cylinder all
responded best to lines that approached the vertical. In fact, a 1-hour
exposure on the 28th day was enough to modify the orientation
selectivity—rapid "entrainment" of multichannel inputs (Blakemore
and Mitchell, 1973; Blakemore, 1974).

Spinelli and his collaborators (1972) allowed six of the kittens
from one of the above experiments normal binocular viewing in an
attempt to determine the possibility and extent of adding other types
of receptive fields by giving other experiences to their visual system.
After exposure to a normal environment for 19 months, it was found
that, indeed, there had been a massive increase in the percentage of
those classes of receptive fields that were either absent or weak at the
end of the selective visual experience. These receptive fields, acquired
during binocular viewing, were often binocular, which apparently is a
critical finding. Another critical observation was that units whose
response characteristics mimic the stimuli viewed during development
were almost completely unchanged, i.e., they were monocularly
activated and had the orientation appropriate for the stimulus viewed
during development by the eye from which they were mapped. Most
impressive are those units whose receptive field shapes are almost a
carbon copy of the three bars viewed during development. *This is 1½
years later and from a single cell!* This study shows that, once cells have
committed themselves to a specific visual feature, they cannot change;
new features seem to be taken up by available, noncommitted cells.

Metzler and Spinelli (1975; Spinelli and Metzler, 1975) tried to
demonstrate that, after differential exposure, horizontal lines appear
"weaker" to the vertically exposed eye and vertical lines appear

"weaker" to the horizontally exposed eye. Accordingly, the cats were trained monocularly to a simple brightness discrimination in a Y-maze. The brighter door could open; both sides were baited with food. After criterion (95% correct trials in the last two sessions) was obtained, catch trials (vertical versus horizontal lines) were randomly inserted. These stimuli, equated for brightness, were generated in order to have the same separation in degree of visual angle, when viewed from the choice point, as the exposure stimuli, when viewed during the 6 weeks of selective exposure. The data show that, when the cats used the vertically exposed eye, they went to the vertical lines almost exclusively, whereas they went to the horizontal lines when using the eye that was exposed to horizontal lines. This effect is interesting in that it was obtained months after the exposure had been terminated and the cats had been allowed normal binocular viewing.

Spinelli and his co-workers (1973) investigated the time course of the plastic changes and their possible reversibility. Kittens were raised in the dark, but they had access to a feeding station. Whenever a kitten went to feed, a picture window lit up that displayed three horizontal bars at a distance of 25 cm. After 13 weeks of exposure, recordings from single cells in the kitten's primary visual cortex showed that all receptive fields were horizontally oriented. Some receptive fields consisted of three excitatory bars separated by the same number of degrees of visual angle as the bars in the stimulus. Further, there was no binocular disparity between the cells, i.e., all receptive fields had perfect correspondence—an important finding in view of our thesis that binocular disparity is the physiological basis for stereoscopy. These results indicate that the basic machinery for vision has to be either built up or exercised very early in life for normal function to be possible in the adult.

Stereopsis: Integrating Theories

Theories of Hysteresis

The Dipole-Array Model

Julesz (1971) has modeled cooperativity in stereopsis using two arrays of magnetic dipoles suspended by ball joints at their center. The model (Figure 36) requires that the dipoles represent cortical units with large receptive fields, and each planar array represents the cortical

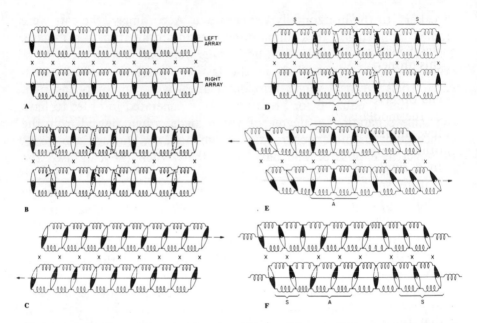

Figure 36. Spring-loaded dipole model under various conditions. A. Entire array is interlocked (fused). B. Uncorrelated arrays attract 50%, repulse 50%. C. Interlocked arrays within the fusional limit. D. Surround is interlocked (fused). E. After surround is interlocked, the center area is aligned and becomes interlocked. F. Refined model in spring-suspended frame; both surround and square have interlocked dipoles. [Julesz, 1971]

mapping of one retina. It is assumed that stimulating the retina is equivalent to orienting the dipoles so that north or south poles turning out from the plane correspond to black and white dots, respectively. Each of the oriented dipoles is spring-coupled to each of its nearest neighbors in the same array. The two arrays representing the mapping from the two retinas are so situated that each of the dipoles in one array is in exact registration with its counterpart in the other array. In such a model the representation of identical retinal stimuli will correspond to a complete alignment of the corresponding dipoles in the two arrays. The interlocking of two dipoles corresponds to local fusion, while the set of all interlocked dipoles corresponds to global fusion. Since local attractions and repulsions will cancel out, the dipole-array representations of uncorrelated patterns will exert no attraction for each other. Disparity of the projections on the two retinas will, after fusion has taken place, yield the angle of orientation of a dipole as an indicator of local depth; this is distinct from the biological reality of different neurons tuned to different disparities. Once the arrays have fused, they can be pulled apart without causing the dipoles to unlock.

In some sense, hyperdipoles have been formed, yielding cooperative stable states. Can the reader think of a morphological machine that has this property?

Analogies between the behavior of the model and the phenomena observed in stereopsis can be pursued further. An interesting aspect of the model is the "search and lock" mechanism. Suppose that only a few dipoles interlock. If the arrays are now shifted relative to each other, more dipoles will be brought into alignment and will interlock. In a similar way in pattern recognition, one can have a search in a feature space and a sequential increase of fusion by the increased number of interlocked features.

One reason why Julesz did not propose a neurophysiological model is obvious. The structure of his dipole model is highly global and no such global disparity units have yet been found by the neurophysiologists. For instance, each of his dipoles corresponds to a hypercomplex disparity unit that integrates the firing of a large number of local disparity units (of the Barlow, Blakemore, and Pettigrew type) that fire for many binocular disparity values but belong to the same, single retinal position. On the other hand, when the springs force many adjacent dipoles to turn together by a constant angle as a hyperdipole, the corresponding hypercomplex neural unit can be regarded as integrating the output of many local binocular disparity cortical units that are tuned to one disparity value but belong to many retinal positions. While the columnar organization of the cortex might suggest extensions of hypercomplex stereopsis units that evaluate the output of local disparity units using a column, it should be stressed that such global units have not yet been found. In the rest of this section we shall study two models, those of Wilson and Cowan (1972) and Dev (1974), that are more closely rooted in neurophysiology.

The Two-Field Model

Wilson and Cowan (1972) have developed a model for the statistical analysis of large-scale interaction of excitatory and inhibitory neurons in a tissue.* Their model is akin to Beurle's (1954, 1956) classic model, save that Wilson and Cowan now pay proper attention to inhibition. The cortex is modeled as a two-dimensional sheet; neurons

---

*This replaces Cowan's earlier attempts to do statistical mechanics by plugging a Hamiltonian description of a network into an ensemble. Cowan is still interested in his even earlier work on reliability and would like to build on it to relate information theory to order-disorder transitions. Furthermore, he believes Marr's (1969) work is valuable at the conceptual level here.

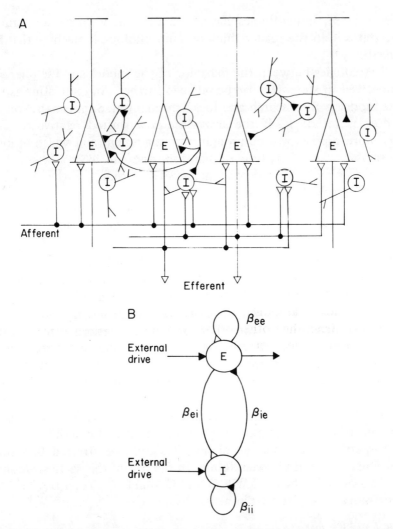

Figure 37. A. Neural tissue comprised of two cell types, E and I, showing recurrent excitation and inhibition. B. The "logic" of A, showing the four types of interaction between the neurons. [Cowan]

are classified as being either excitatory, e.g., Golgi type I cells, or inhibitory, e.g., interneurons (Figure 37A). Since the states of the two neuronal populations must be described separately, a minimal model is a two-field model in which there is no further subdivision of the excitatory and inhibitory populations. The activity in such a field is characterized by the fraction of excitatory neurons becoming active per unit time, $P_e(t)$, and the corresponding fraction of activated inhibitory neurons, $P_i(t)$. The four types of interconnections (Figure 37B) are represented by the functions $\beta_{ee}(x)$, $\beta_{ei}(x)$, $\beta_{ie}(x)$, and $\beta_{ii}(x)$, where e represents an excitatory neuron and i, an inhibitory neuron. Each interconnection function depends exponentially on the ratio of the separation $(x - x_0)$ between the interacting neurons to the characteristic space constant σ. Thus, for example, for the inhibition exerted on excitatory cells, the connection function is

$$\beta_{ie}(x) = e^{|x - x_0|/\sigma_{ie}} \tag{1}$$

It is assumed that the inhibitory interconnections are longer than their excitatory counterparts; thus the fields have an excitatory center and inhibitory surround organization. It is also assumed that the population of cells has a Gaussian distribution of threshold. Neural activation as a function of intensity of input is described by a sigmoid curve, which always turns up in cooperative phenomena and is responsible for hysteresis.

Time-averaging the activity in this abstraction of cortical tissue yields a model in the form of a pair of coupled nonlinear integrodifferential equations for the state functions characterizing the activity of large groups of neurons. By solving the system of equations for different values of the connectivity parameters, three different dynamic modes are observed: (1) active transient response, (2) limit-cycle oscillations, and (3) spatially inhomogeneous, stable steady states.

In the active transient mode, the response to a localized stimulus continues to increase and reaches its peak value after the stimulus has ceased. Only for stimuli of sufficiently long duration is the threshold reached for this effect, i.e., temporal summation is involved in reaching the threshold. Another generic property of the tissue characteristic of the active transient mode is edge-enhancement in response to wide stimuli, and associated with this property is a latency.

One can see the similarity of this system of equations to the Lotka-Volterra equations where the excitatory and inhibitory populations correspond to predator and prey, respectively. Indeed, in the second dynamic form of the solution, the oscillation is like that in population dynamics; the response to a constant stimulus consists of limit-cycle oscillations (see Katchalsky et al., 1974). (Compare the Andersen and Eccles model (1962) of thalamic relay nuclei.) For a periodic input, the response may be frequency demultiplication.

The activity in a sheet of tissue can be synchronized or desynchronized by inhibition or disinhibition from another sheet of tissue. Such inhibitory afferents affect extensive regions in a diffuse manner. If, for example, strong diffuse inhibition (to the inhibitory neurons) is superimposed on spatially patterned excitation (to the excitatory neurons), a new form of solution evolves, consisting of a pair of waves propagating from the point of excitation with a velocity on the order of centimeters per second (cf. Burns's (1968) experiments on undercut cortex).

The third mode of the solution consists of spatially inhomogeneous, stable steady states. The neuronal activity, once initiated, is self-maintained. This may result from the reverberation of signals due to strong recurrent excitation. Wilson and Cowan suggest that the active transient mode may be characteristic of the primary sensory cortex, particularly the visual cortex. They find support for this in the observation that the model can simulate characteristics of various psychophysical phenomena. When the excitatory neurons are stimulated with spatially varying stimuli, the transfer function of the tissue model exhibits attenuation at both low and high spatial frequencies, in a manner characteristic of the visual system. With this model, one can also simulate backward masking and a hysteresis response to a pair of point stimuli akin to that seen by Fender and Julesz (1967) in binocular vision. In the simulation, hysteresis is observed when the distance between peaks of excitatory neuronal activity is plotted against the distance between peak amplitudes of the stimuli. A purely excitatory system can exhibit a simple hysteresis, whereas one with both excitation and inhibition can show a complex hysteresis. However, Julesz expressed scepticism about comparisons between his dipole model and that of Wilson and Cowan, since the latter is inherently a monocular model. The search and lock feature of the Julesz dipole model (and the hysteresis between interlocked left and right arrays) is very different from the hysteresis effect in a single array used by Wilson and Cowan.

Figure-Ground Separation Model

The second neurophysiological approach is afforded by the Dev (1974) model of figure-ground separation, which can be applied to the psychological data provided by Julesz' studies on the perception of random-dot stereograms (see Figure 38). Since the input to each eye is a random pattern, monocular input carries no information. Interesting information is *only* contained in the correlation between the two patterns. Substantial regions of both patterns are identical in appearance and location; other regions are identical in appearance but are

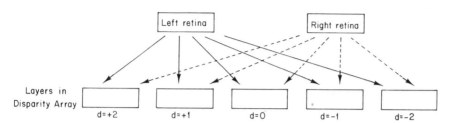

Figure 38. A model for the stereoscopic perception of surfaces at different depths from the observer. The left and right retinas project to the five layers in the disparity array with the output of the right retina being shifted laterally by an amount d with respect to that of the left retina. [Dev]

laterally displaced. This lateral displacement results in a perception of depth, and the visual system is able to detect these displacements or disparities by a comparison of the two patterns. If the comparison requires perception of many regions of different disparities, the subject may take seconds to perceive the stereogram. During this time the subjective reports will be of periods in which no change is perceived, followed by the sudden emergence of yet another surface from the pattern of random dots.

To clarify the concept of ambiguity of disparity in Julesz' stereograms, turn to the linear arrays of Figure 39 (Arbib et al., 1974). The top two lines illustrate the pattern of random input to the two eyes. The numbers 1 and 0 correspond to the presence or absence of a dot, respectively, at that location. The top line shows the 21 randomly generated 0's and 1's (or bits) that constitute the "left-eye input," while the second line is the "right-eye input" obtained by displacing the

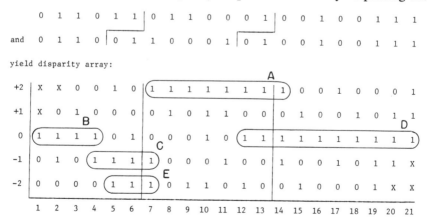

Figure 39. The problem of resolving ambiguity. [Arbib et al., 1974]

pattern at locations 7 through 13 two places left (so that the bit at position i goes to position $i - 2$ for $7 \leqslant i \leqslant 13$), while the bits at positions 12 and 13 thus left vacant are filled in at random. In the remaining 5 lines of Figure 39, a disparity array with 5 layers is shown. The disparity of the ith bit in line d is a 1 if the ith bit of the right-eye input equals the $(i + d)$th bit of the left-eye input.

The disparity array of Figure 39 suggests a stripped-down caricature of the visual cortex. Rather than mimic a columnar organization, the model segregates the mock cortex into layers. The initial activity of a cell in position i of layer d corresponds to the occurrence of a match between the activity of cell i of the right retina and cell $(i + d)$ of the left retina.* (This positioning of the elements aids our conceptualization. It is not the *positioning* of neurons that should be subject to experimental test, but rather the relationships posited between them.) As shown in Figure 39, the initial activity in these layers indicates both the "true" correlations (A signals the central "surface"; B and D signal the "background") and the "spurious" signals (the clumps of activity at C and E in addition to the scattered 1's, resulting from the probability of ½ that a random pair of bits will match), which obscure the true correlations.

Can the neurons of the disparity array be interconnected in such a way that the spurious correlations, including the activity at C and E, are suppressed? We might imagine (but only as a crude first approximation) the resultant activity in the disparity array, localized in regions A, B, and D, as providing a suitable input for a higher level, pattern-recognition device that can in some way recognize the three-dimensional object whose visible surfaces have been so clearly represented in the brain.

The aim, then, is to divide the visual field (whose spatial extent is indicated by the numbers 1 through $n = 21$) into a number of regions so that in each region only cells of one layer of the disparity array are active. The spatial extent of the regions, k in number, can be indicated by $(1, x_1)$, (x_1, x_2), ... (x_{k-1}, n), where $x_1, x_2, \ldots x_{k-1}$ are the boundaries between the regions. In dividing the visual field, we are guided by the plausible hypothesis—stressed above—that our visual world is made up of relatively few connected regions. The "optimization principle" will, therefore, attempt to choose the boundaries between the regions, $x_1, x_2, \ldots x_{k-1}$, in such a way as to minimize k

---

*i indicates the position in an array and may have values from 1 to 21. d indicates the layer within the disparity array and has values from +2 to −2.

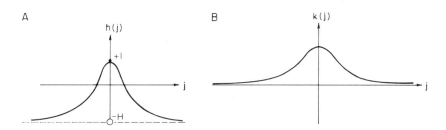

Figure 40. The functions for (A) inhibitory interaction of layers and (B) excitatory interaction of neighboring cells in Dev's segmentation model. $h(j)$ and $k(j)$ are the interconnection functions between neurons. H is a constant. [Arbib et al., 1974]

while at the same time accounting for most of the original activity in the array. The optimization is achieved by the use of a simple interconnection scheme that yields qualitatively appropriate behavior of the disparity array without directly minimizing k.

The essential interconnection is given by the following rules: (1) there should be moderate, local cross-excitation within a layer of the disparity array and (2) inhibition between layers should increase as the difference in disparity increases. Let $x_{di}(t)$ represent the activity of the cell at position i in layer d at time t, and let the interconnection functions, $h(j)$ and $k(j)$, be represented by the form indicated by Figure 40. Then, the change of activity in a cell is given in the model by the following equation:

$$x_{di}(t+1) = \Sigma_{d'}\Sigma_{i'}h(d-d')k(i-i')x_{d'i'}(t) + x_{di}^{0} \qquad (2)$$

where the value of x is not permitted to exceed 1 or drop below 0.

The connectivity scheme allows a cluster of active cells in one layer to suppress scattered activity of cells in other layers in the same region, while simultaneously facilitating the activity of neighboring cells in their own layer. Eventually, the system reaches a state in which the activity is segregated into clearly defined regions in different layers without spatial overlap between any of those regions. Since, in any region, activity is restricted to a single layer, there is no ambiguity of disparity information. Moreover, the dynamics of the model represent the phenomenon of the time lag and the abrupt perception of surfaces that occurs during observation of Julesz' random-dot stereograms. This is simulated in the model by the fact that, once a cluster of activity reaches a critical size, it will then spread rapidly to form almost its final size.

Another aspect of this simple model that should be noted is that Equation 2 can be rewritten in a fashion that suggests a plausible scheme of neural interconnection. If the neurons of the disparity array are excitatory and a layer of inhibitory interneurons is now introduced, the activity of the ith inhibitory interneuron at time t is given by the simple equation

$$y_i(t) = \Sigma_d x_{di}(t) \tag{3}$$

A constant, H, can be selected so that for all j's

$$\bar{h}(j) = H + h(j) \geqslant 0 \tag{4}$$

Equation 2 can be rewritten as

$$x_{di}(t + 1) = \Sigma_{d'}\Sigma_{i'}(\bar{h}(d - d') - H)k(i - i')x_{d'i'}(t) + x_{di}^0 \tag{5}$$

so that

$$x_{di}(t + 1) = \left\{\Sigma_{d'}\Sigma_{i'}\bar{h}(d - d')k(i - i')x_{d'i'}(t)\right\} - \Sigma_{i'}\ell(i - i')y_{i'}(t) + x_{di}^0 \tag{6}$$

where $\ell(i - i') = Hk(i - i')$. Thus, Equation 6 shows that the model may be given structural expression in a form in which *the x_{di} are all excitatory, with excitation decreasing with distance and being appropriately counteracted by a single layer of inhibitory interneurons.*

The resultant architecture of several layers of excitatory neurons interacting with each other and with a single layer of inhibitory neurons may be regarded as a natural generalization of the Wilson-Cowan (1972) scheme of interaction of a single excitatory layer with a layer of inhibitory interneurons. A similar procedure has been used by Wässle and Creutzfeldt (1973) for simulating receptive fields and two-line discrimination of retinal and geniculate neurons, and by Malsburg (1973) for simulating an orientation-sensitive cortical network.

V. CEREBELLAR FUNCTION

Our ideas on the role of the cerebellum in the control of movement have been shaped by clinical data on movement abnormality in patients with cerebellar lesions. A classic example is that of Holmes (1939): a subject can form smooth alternating movements with the hand on the side with a normal cerebellum, whereas on the side with cerebellar lesions the hand movements are dysmetric, i.e., inaccurate and jerky (Figure 41). In this chapter, we probe the detailed mechanisms that enable the cerebellum to play the role of modulator of movement suggested by the clinical data.

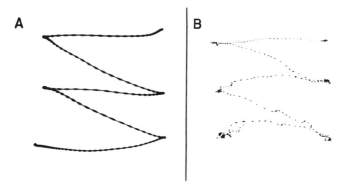

Figure 41. Normal (A) and dysmetric (B) movements of a hand whose ipsilateral cerebellum is normal (A) and destroyed by gunshot wounds (B). [Holmes, 1939]

The Basic Circuitry of the Cerebellar Cortex

Although some aspects of cerebellar circuitry are discussed in Chapter III, in this section we present not only a more comprehensive view of that circuitry but also its relation to three models of the cerebellar cortex. The basic neuronal connections of the cerebellar cortex are summarized in Figure 42A, which shows that there are only two kinds of afferent fibers conveying information to the cortex of the cerebellum, the climbing fibers (CF) and the mossy fibers (MF), whereas there is only one type of efferent fiber from the cerebellum, the axons of the Purkinje cells (PC). These axons terminate in the cerebellar nuclei (CN). The climbing fiber exerts a powerful excitatory action on a single Purkinje cell, yielding the typical climbing fiber

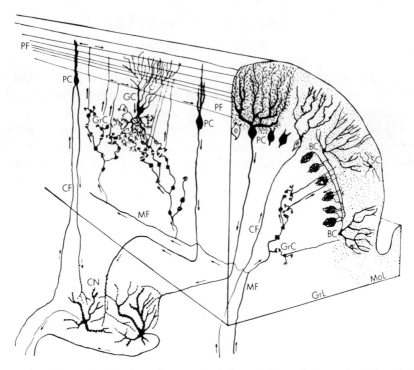

Figure 42A. Perspective drawing of a part of a folium of the cerebellar cortex. The principal components are shown in diagrammatic form. BC = basket cell; CF = climbing fiber; CN = cerebellar nuclei; GrC = granule cell; GrL = granular layer; MF = mossy fiber; MoL = molecular layer; PC = Purkinje cell; PF = parallel fiber; SC = stellate cell. [Adapted from Fox, 1962]

response (CFr), i.e., a burst of up to 4 or 5 spikes. However, it should be stressed for later reference that the CFr is followed by an inactivation of the Purkinje cell (Granit and Phillips, 1956). On the other hand, the mossy fiber input, which is characterized by an enormous divergence, exerts (via interneurons) both excitatory and inhibitory actions on Purkinje cells. The excitatory pathway is by mossy fibers to granule cells (GrC) that discharge impulses along their axons; these branch to form the parallel fibers (PF) that give excitatory synapses to Purkinje cells. The inhibitory pathway is by mossy fibers to granule cells to parallel fibers to basket cells (BC) that project a dense array of inhibitory synapses on the bodies of the Purkinje cells. The approximate divergence and convergence numbers are given in Figure 42B.

As shown in Figure 42C, cerebellar circuitry exhibits both feedback and feedforward inhibition: inhibitory feedforward mechanisms are mediated by the basket cell synapses on Purkinje cells and by Purkinje cell output on the cerebellar nuclei, whereas the inhibitory feedback loop is from granule cell to Golgi cell and back to granule cell.

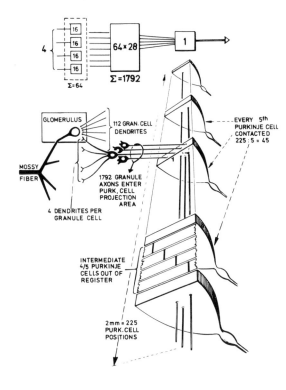

Figure 42B. Block diagram at top shows the total numerical transfer in the mossy fiber-Purkinje cell neuron chain. Diagram at bottom is intended to give a comprehensive idea of the numerical and metrical relations of the neuron chain with the essential data indicated. For simplicity, granule cell axons are shown to enter the surface projection area of the Purkinje cells from above, whereas in reality they enter from below. Number of parallel fibers crossing Purkinje dendritic tree = 225 × 1792 ~ 400,000; calculated number of synapses = 400,000 ÷ 5 = 80,000; counted number of spines = 91,000. [Palkovits et al., 1972]

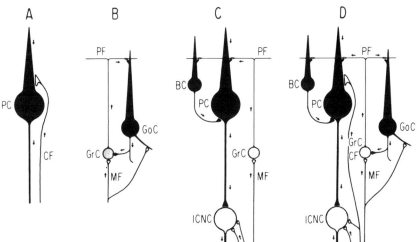

Figure 42C. The most significant cells and their synaptic connections in the cerebellar cortex. The component circuits of *A*, *B*, and *C* are assembled together in *D*. Arrows show lines of operation; inhibitory cells are solid. BC = basket cell; CF = climbing fiber; GoC = Golgi cell; GrC = granule cell; ICNC = intracerebellar nuclear cell; MF = mossy fiber; PC = Purkinje cell; PF = parallel fiber. [Eccles, 1973b]

Mossy Fiber Action

The mossy fiber action is effected in the rectangular lattice that is principally determined by the parallel course of the parallel fibers for about 2 mm along a cerebellar folium and by the basket cell axons that spread for 0.6 mm perpendicular to the parallel fibers. A sharply focused mossy fiber input would give a "beam" of parallel fiber impulses that results in a 2-mm strip of excited Purkinje cells "on-beam," and, by action of the basket cells, a zone of inhibited Purkinje cells 0.6 mm "off-beam" on either side (Figure 43).

However, this notion is too schematic in view of the fact that input to the cerebellum is not confined to a few beams of mossy fiber activation. The diverse activity of even closely neighboring Purkinje cells, which was noticed independently by Eccles and his collaborators (1971c) and by Llinás and his co-workers (1971) at about the same

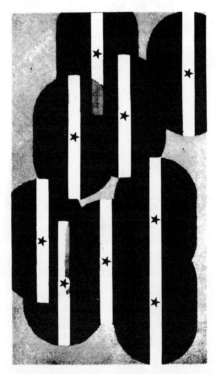

Figure 43. Illustration of the interaction on Purkinje cells of excitation provided by parallel fibers and of inhibition produced by lateral inhibition of basket cells for nine focused mossy fiber inputs (stars). The overlapping excitatory strips with inhibitory surrounds result in a pattern of various levels of Purkinje cell excitation, as indicated by the shading. [Eccles, 1973b]

time, should also be stressed. At the Work Session, Eccles commented that the Purkinje cell responses are, indeed, much more individualized than would have been anticipated from the extensive branching of a single mossy fiber and of the further distribution of mossy fiber activity via parallel fibers and basket cells.

This picture becomes less mysterious in light of the new structural analysis of the cerebellar network by Palkovits and his colleagues (1971a,b,c, 1972), demonstrating the staggered position of neighboring Purkinje cells relative to the parallel fiber direction and also the relatively few synapses formed between the parallel fibers and the Purkinje cell dendritic trees that the fibers cross (see Figure 16). Clearly, one needs no longer to assume that neighboring Purkinje cells in the longitudinal direction of the folium would be stimulated under similar circumstances.

In view of this complexity, computer simulation is required to chart the effect of a widely distributed mossy fiber input. Pellionisz and Szentágothai (1974) simulated a model of the cerebellar cortex consisting of stacked two-dimensional neuron matrices with two emerging and subsiding foci of mossy fiber input in close proximity. This simulation, in which the effects of the spatiotemporal patterns of parallel fiber activation on Purkinje dendrites have also been considered, gives a vivid picture of the integration of neighboring foci. Closely spaced Purkinje cells show individual behavior within the zones where the border of the foci are merging: some cells being driven by one focus, some by the other, and a third group by both foci. This occurs even in a "basic circuit" without the inhibitory systems of Golgi and basket cells.

The spatiotemporal aspects of this neighborhood relation, however, are greatly modified and improved by introducing the Golgi and basket cell systems: the Golgi cell feedback improves the integration of the foci by enlarging their overlap and produces a speed-up response of Purkinje cells with increased phasic character. Conversely, basket cell feedforward inhibition provides a spatial *and* temporal separation of the integrative activity from the neighboring foci. In space, this occurs not only as lateral inhibition, but also as longitudinal (parallel fiber) inhibition, whereas in the time domain, by delaying the response of foci, the integrative activity is neatly separated.

The secondary improving effects of the inhibitory systems on the basic mechanism can best be shown in the simulated functioning of the faulty network model of the cerebellar cortex of immobilized kittens. As already mentioned in Chapter III, if a kitten is raised in wax boots with lead weights, the animal grows up ataxic. Examination of the cerebellum shows that the number of spines per Purkinje cell is the same, but the parallel fibers are shorter than those of a normal kitten. Therefore, the synapses must be closer. Thus, in a kitten raised in a restricted environment, a number of wrong synaptic connections are made. The simulation shows that, with these shorter parallel fibers, the integration of the foci is seriously affected in the basic circuit, whereas with the help of the Golgi and basket cell systems it can be improved considerably.

Braitenberg's Timing Model

The first theory of the cerebellum to take account of the lattice geometry of the cerebellar cortex was formulated by Braitenberg (1961, 1967a, 1973; Braitenberg and Atwood, 1958; Braitenberg and Onesto, 1960). The theory's most general assertion, that timing in the millisecond range must be important in the cerebellum, has already entered neurological literature to such a degree as to seem obvious; it has also received some support from Freeman (1969).

Other mechanisms suggested by Braitenberg have been recently discussed by Kornhuber (1971). For a clearer picture of these mechanisms, it is worth making some observations on the ballistic movements of an animal's limbs, as in the following example. When a shot is fired from a gun, two pulsatile forces are involved: the explosion that propels the projectile towards the target and the braking force that results when the projectile hits the target. If the target were to step aside, the projectile would not stop in the position at which it was originally aimed. The ballistic movements of an animal's limbs also involve a similar "bang-bang" control for starting and stopping the movement. There is (1) an initial acceleration of the limb as the agonist muscles contract and the antagonist muscles relax, (2) an intervening quiet period, and then (3) the final deceleration as the antagonist muscles contract. Experiments on rapid flexion and extension of joints have shown that muscle activation occupies only a small portion of the movement, and that the duration of this activation does not seem to be related to the extent of the movement. Thus, the duration of the movement seems to be determined mainly by the timing of the "stop" signal. This timing has to be determined by the brain rather than be imposed by the environment, as in the projectile example.

Braitenberg proposed an elegant network for converting space into time by providing that the position of an input to the cerebellar cortex (encoding the desired target position) would determine the time of the output (which would stop the movement by activating the antagonist muscles). The scheme has a linear array of Purkinje cells whose output circuitry is so arranged that the firing of any one of them will yield the antagonist burst that will "brake" the ballistic movement. There are two systems of inputs to these Purkinje cells, the mossy fibers and the climbing fibers, each arranged in a linear array. The position of each fiber in the array corresponds to an angle of flexion of the joint. Each climbing fiber connects to a single Purkinje cell. The mossy fibers contact granule cells whose axons bifurcate, forming parallel fibers that contact each Purkinje cell in the array. The speed of propagation along the parallel fibers of this model is such that the time required to go from one point to another in the array corresponds to the time required by the joint to move between the corresponding angles.

The command system in this model was posited to elicit a ballistic movement of a limb by firing three signals: one signal to trigger the burst in the agonist muscles initiating movement, another to the climbing fiber corresponding to the initial joint position,* and a third signal to the mossy fiber corresponding to the target position of the limb. If we assume that a Purkinje cell can respond to parallel fiber input only if it has also received climbing fiber input, then the Purkinje cell activated will be the one whose climbing fiber is active. Furthermore, the time of firing of the Purkinje cell will correspond to its distance from the activated mossy fiber. Thus, it will elicit the braking effect of the antagonist burst at precisely the right time. Owing to the detailed discoveries concerning the neurophysiology of cerebellar neurons, the original theory is no longer easily and directly applicable to the cortex. Nonetheless, the splendid ideas about timing that it proposes remain among the most stimulating in the history of cerebellar modeling.

Marr's Learning Model

In contrast, Marr (1969), in his model of the cerebellar cortex, incorporated many detailed findings of Eccles and his collaborators

---

*The command system can be relieved of having to "know" where the joint is by having a feedback circuit continually monitor joint position and keep the appropriate climbing fiber activated.

(1967), but his resultant model of cerebellar learning seems (at least to the authors of this *Bulletin*) further removed from the role of the cerebellum in movement than Braitenberg's theory. Despite our skepticism as to the value of Marr's theory as a model of the cerebellar cortex per se, it should be regarded as a valuable addition to the armament with which the theorist may attack the complexity and diversity of neural networks. The theory has two components: The better-known first component views the Purkinje cell as a trainable device that can be triggered by its climbing fiber to yield a signal that elicits an "elemental movement." The pattern of parallel fiber activation impinging upon the Purkinje cell at that time is taken to encode the "context" in which the movement was elicited. By strengthening a parallel fiber synapse whenever climbing fiber activity coincides with activation of that parallel fiber,* the cell can be trained to respond to parallel fiber input alone. Having "learned" the context in which its elemental movement should be elicited, the Purkinje cell can be activated by appropriate mossy fiber input without its climbing fiber trigger. As the second component of his theory (which may prove more widely applicable to neural network theory than the better-known learning component), Marr introduces the notion of a *codon* as a subset of mossy fibers whose co-activation encodes an afferent input event. He points out that, as the overall level of mossy fiber activity increases, the codons may become overloaded, but that the Golgi cells may function as codon-size regulators by providing extra inhibition at the glomeruli (mossy fiber → granule cell synapses).

Cowan related Marr's study to the Winograd and Cowan (1963) model of reliable computation in the presence of noise in the following way: Suppose we are interested in how a computer designer can obtain a reliable computer using cheap components and poor connectivity. (This approach is the opposite of Marr's, who has a perfect computer but ambiguous and complex stimuli.) The fundamental theorem of Winograd and Cowan shows that reliability can be obtained by enlarging the ensemble-distributing structure among functions, and function among structures. Reliability of computation is increased (1) by increasing the number of times a function is carried out, (2) by computing many different functions of a subset of inputs, and (3) by choosing random subsets of inputs. In other words, first a disjunctive analysis of the inputs is carried out, followed by a conjunction of the

---

*The reader may wish to compare this with the perceptron scheme of Rosenblatt (1957); for an exposition, see Nilsson (1965).

results. Cowan suggested that this use of a nonlocal representation would allow one to relate Marr's codons to the fundamental theorem of coding theory. He also stressed that in any model of neural activity the key concepts are distributed computation, multiple representation, and stored programs.

Interestingly, current computer design does not use redundancy at the hardware level. It is perhaps worth adding that Cowan's reliable computer (and Marr's theory) uses binary switching and nonbrain-like assumptions, such as each bit of information being equally valuable and the order of the bits being unimportant. If we turn to more realistic systems, even the primary fact of spatial overlap of receptive fields gives some reliability.

During the discussion of these models, Boylls noted that Marr's trainability theory of the cerebellum implies that climbing fibers are not necessary in the adult cerebellum. Hence, a lesion in the olive should cause no cerebellar deficit in automatic actions. However, the findings of Murphy and O'Leary (1971) do show such deficits. Julesz added that, in an age of computers, where any visual stimulus can be generated, an attempt should be made to define the elemental movements. In his laboratory, they are using infrared techniques to record eye movements during ocular tracking of moving dots and to generate real time movies that are coupled to eye movements (Julesz, 1971).* It would be interesting to observe the behavior of patients with cerebellar lesions and to generate elemental movements with such techniques.

Feedback and Feedforward in Cerebellar Control

An interesting attempt to use the concepts of feedback and feedforward (see Chapter II) has been made by Ito (1970, 1972a,b, 1974) in his study of the vestibulocerebellum. The vestibular organ participates in two major reflexes: the vestibulospinal reflex (VSR) that maintains a steady head position despite body movements, and the vestibuloocular reflex (VOR) that holds the retinal image steady during head movement. The VSR is a closed loop system. The vestibular organ senses head movements and uses negative feedback to correct for head displacement (Figure 44). The VOR, on the other hand, is open loop in

*B. Julesz and W. J. Kropfl, manuscript in preparation.

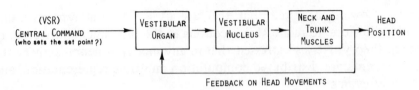

Figure 44. In the vestibulospinal reflex (VSR) the vestibular organ senses head movements and uses negative feedback to correct for head displacement. [Arbib and Szentágothai]

its action. The vestibular organ detects head movement and causes a compensatory eye movement so as to hold the retinal image steady. However, there is no feedback to ensure that the retinal image is indeed held steady. Ito suggests that the cerebellum provides the feedforward tuning for the VOR, and that cerebellar function is modifiable via visual feedback. In the VOR, as in the VSR, the feedforward control can solve loop-time problems in quick movements. A more detailed view of the VOR is provided in Figure 45, which shows the flocculus receiving the same primary vestibular afferent signals that are fed to the secondary vestibular neurons. The output of the flocculus affects three of the four groups of secondary vestibular neurons.

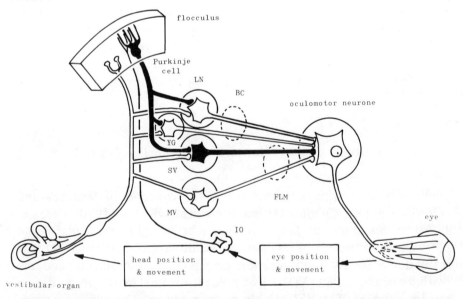

Figure 45. Neuronal connection between the vestibuloocular reflex arc and the flocculus. BC = brachium conjunctivum; FLM = fasciculus longitudinalis medialis; IO = inferior olive; LN = cerebellar lateral nucleus; MV = medial vestibular nucleus; SV = superior vestibular nucleus; YG = the *y* group of the vestibular nuclear complex. Inhibitory neurons are solid; excitatory neurons are open. [Ito, 1974]

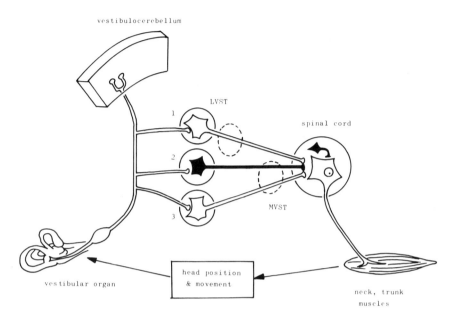

Figure 46A. Neuronal construction of the vestibulospinal reflex arc. LVST = lateral vestibulospinal tract; MVST = medial vestibulospinal tract; 1 = fast excitatory LVST cell; 2 = slow
inhibitory MVST cell; 3 = fast excitatory MVST cell. [Ito, 1974]

Ito speculates that learning based on visual feedback might
improve cerebellar feedforward control of the VOR. (Floccular lesions
yield a phase delay in eye holding during head movement.) He points
out that Lorente de Nó (1931) found that rabbits exhibit a poor VOR
before opening their eyes, but showed an accurate VOR by 40 days,
with vision playing a role in its development. In their recent study of
the effects of protracted use of inverting prisms on the VOR, Gonshor
and Melvill Jones (1973) found that after 5 days the VOR disappeared
and that thereafter it occurred with reversed polarity. After removal of
the prisms, 4 weeks were required to restore the VOR to normal.
Although there is no evidence of cerebellar involvement in this learning,
Ito, bearing in mind the work of Marr (1969) mentioned above, still
finds this idea attractive. Noting that VOR learning takes many days, he
wonders whether cerebellar learning is too slow for acute experiments.

In the VSR circuitry (Figure 46A), the secondary sensory cell
groups have been categorized into three types: (1) those with lateral
vestibular tract axons conducting with a relatively fast velocity and
exerting an excitatory action upon spinal neurons, (2) those with
inhibitory and slowly conducting medial vestibular tract axons, and

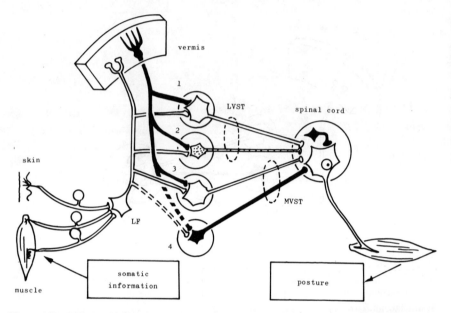

Figure 46B. Relationship between the spinovestibulospinal reflex arc and the cerebellar vermis. LF = spinocerebellar afferents ascending through the lateral funiculus, 1 = fast excitatory LVST cell; 2 = slow LVST cell with unknown synaptic action; 3 = fast excitatory MVST cell; 4 = slow inhibitory MVST cell. Interrupted lines indicate uncertainty for the connections to group 4 neuron. [Ito, 1974]

(3) those with excitatory and fast-conducting medial vestibular tract axons. These three types are free from Purkinje cell inhibition. Further, control does not seem to require the assistance of the spinal cord. However, somatic information also feeds these three groups as well as a fourth (inhibitory action) group (Figure 46B), and the Purkinje cells of vermis do have an inhibitory influence on all four types. These findings support the idea of a somatic feedforward effect in posture, e.g., the tonic neck reflex. (There is some overlap of VOR and VSR with some vestibular neurons serving both arcs.)

In the rabbit, Maekawa and Simpson (1972, 1973) found that visual information passes via the midbrain (central tegmental tract and accessory optic tract (AOT)) to the inferior olive and thence to the flocculus via the climbing fibers.* There is a 10-msec latency from the

*At the 1972 NRP Third Study Program in Boulder, Colorado, W.J.H. Nauta commented that the AOT → inferior olive path was a surprise since the AOT and its nuclei have been suggested to convey retinal impulses to the pineal gland by way of the peripheral sympathetic. Ito replied that Simpson excluded an effect of the visual cortex on climbing fiber input to the flocculus, but found that stimulation of the accessory optic nucleus yielded a dramatic climbing fiber effect that was not affected by ablation of the visual cortex or superior colliculus and appeared to be transmitted through the central tegmentum.

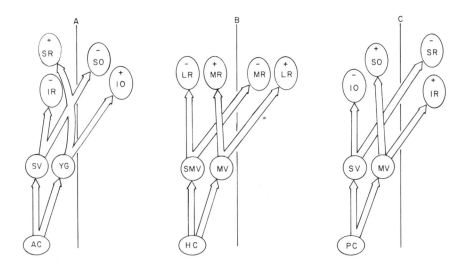

Figure 47. Principal pathways of vestibuloocular reflexes. AC = anterior canal; HC = horizontal canal; IO = inferior oblique; IR = inferior rectus; LR = lateral rectus; MR = medial rectus; MV = medial vestibular nucleus; PC = posterior canal; SMV = superior vestibular nucleus and medial vestibular nucleus; SO = superior oblique; SR = superior rectus; SV = superior vestibular nucleus; YG = group *y*. –, inhibitory action; +, excitatory action. [Ito, 1973]

optic tract to the flocculus, of which 4 msec is from the inferior olive to the flocculus (the rabbit retina imposes a 40-msec delay). The climbing fiber response is from *ipsilateral* optic stimulation. Maekawa and Natsui (1973) found the floccular cells of the rabbit to be along the long, horizontal foveal line, with the preferred stimulus being a vertical slit moving horizontally. They observed a few horizontal receptive fields but no oblique ones, suggesting that the floccular Purkinje cells are monitoring eye movements rather than recognizing patterns.

Each of the two vestibular organs provides five types of input: the anterior, horizontal, and posterior canals are velocity sensors; the utricle and saccule indicate head position relative to the vertical. There are twelve groups of oculomotoneurons corresponding to the six muscle groups for each eye. Of the 120 (10 vestibular input × 12 oculomotor output) possible connections, Ito has found the specific connections shown in Figure 47, which are essentially the same as those already deduced from anatomical studies (Szentágothai, 1943) and subsequently shown physiologically by Szentágothai (1950, 1952b). The vertical line indicates the animal's midline and shows that paired relaxation occurs: each canal yields inhibition of one member and excitation of the other member of an agonist-antagonist pair.

Floccular stimulation does serve to repress oculomotor response to vestibular stimulation. However, as schematized in Figure 48 for the

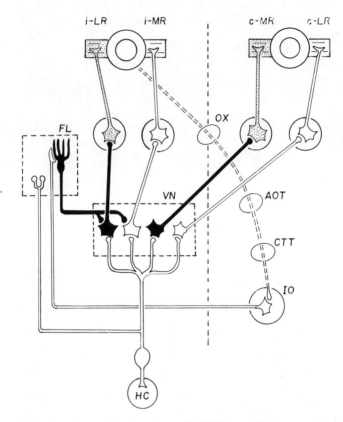

Figure 48. Schematic drawing showing that only half the oculomotor pathways are under floccular control. AOT = accessory optical tract; CTT = central tegmental tract; c-MR = contralateral medial rectus; c-LR = contralateral lateral rectus; FL = flocculus; HC = horizontal canal; i-LR = ipsilateral lateral rectus; i-MR = ipsilateral medial rectus; IO = inferior olive; OX = optic chiasm; VN = vestibular nucleus. [Ito, 1973]

horizontal eye-movement system, only half the pathways (the ipsi-lateral ones) are under floccular control. Each eye muscle receives two vestibular inputs, one excitatory and one inhibitory, and only one of each pair is under floccular control; thus, the flocculus is not "fighting itself."

According to Boylls,* Ito's results provide a fresh look at the role of climbing fibers. Although their synapses on cerebellar Purkinje neurons are physiologically excitatory, the assumption that these fibers provoke augmented inhibition upon target cerebellar and vestibular nuclear cells is questionable, owing to the climbing fiber "inactivation response" (see above) and the climbing fiber collateral excitation of

*C. C. Boylls, personal communication.

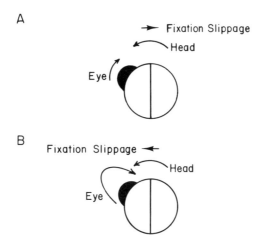

Figure 49. A. VOR gain insufficient. B. VOR gain excessive. The VOR to identical, ipsilateral head rotations under two different gain conditions, yielding two cases of fixation slippage. Only the ipsilateral eye is shown (see the text). [Boylls, 1975]

cerebellar nuclear neurons. These observations might be simply (though not exclusively) incorporated into a story of concomitant Purkinje cell depression. To relate this to the above discussion, Boylls first noted that, according to Ito's hypotheses, the climbing fibers of Figure 48 adjust VOR gain by altering the level of flocculus inhibition upon the vestibular nuclei. If one makes the further assumption that the flocculus on one side of the midline controls the VOR for head movements *only* towards that side (since such turns excite the ipsilateral horizontal canal), the effects of climbing fiber input on the VOR can be deduced from the visually evoked responses in the climbing fibers.

In examining Figure 49, note that both the upper and lower portions of the figure portray an identical, horizontal ipsilateral head rotation and simultaneous VOR in the ipsilateral eye, but under two different gain conditions. In Figure 49A, the gain is insufficient; the opposing eye rotation is less than that of the head. As a result, the fixated visual field "slips" in the caudocranial (posterior-to-anterior) direction. Likewise, in Figure 49B, the VOR gain is excessive, causing too great an eye rotation and visual slippage craniocaudally. According to the previous hypotheses, then, caudocranial slippage in these rotations must indicate *excessive* floccular inhibition, while craniocaudal sliding betrays the reverse. The question is: "If the climbing fibers secure adjustments in this inhibition, to which type of slippage do they respond?"

As mentioned above, floccular climbing fibers respond very well to moving visual stimuli, usually to vertical bars moving horizontally (Maekawa and Natsui, 1973); however, directional sensitivity is not yet definitively reported. Simpson and Alley (1973), though, have described a general caudocranial preference of nodular climbing fibers, and Ito (1974) has reported unpublished work of Maekawa indicating a similar observation in flocculus. If the floccular climbing fibers are eventually found distinctively excitable by caudocranially moving visual targets—and if the assumptions given above are correct—this would provide strong indirect evidence for a long-term depressive influence of climbing fiber input upon Purkinje cell inhibition. Alternatively, the climbing fibers could be viewed as enhancing the outflow from the entire cerebellar nuclear complex.

It should be noted that Ito (1974) has observed a brief depression of vestibular canal-induced eye muscle contraction following climbing fiber activation from the visual pathway. If, however, climbing fibers serve to produce gradual, extended alterations in cerebellar activity, possibly through repeated activation, then experimentation should not be confined solely to the first 100 msec or so following the stimulus. For example, to secure a 25% alteration in the human VOR through visual feedback (and thus possible climbing fiber mediation) requires about 1 hour (Gonshor and Melvill Jones, 1973). How does the VOR respond to frequent climbing fiber stimuli over such intervals?

In summary, Boylls has suggested a method for deducing floccular climbing fiber influences on the VOR from their visual properties. The method is based upon the following assumptions: (1) the ipsilateral flocculus governs by inhibition the positional gain of the VOR to ipsilateral, horizontal head rotations, and (2) the climbing fibers adjust this inhibition pursuant to conditions of fixation slippage symptomatic of various VOR gain settings. It may be that this method will yield behavioral evidence showing a net depressive effect of climbing fibers on floccular inhibition, or a like augmentation of outflow from the cerebellar (and vestibular) nuclei.

Cerebrocerebellar Interactions

It is now appropriate to turn from this elegant scheme of oculomotor control to a consideration of Eccles' views on the cerebellar involvement in the spinal control of limb movement and its integration

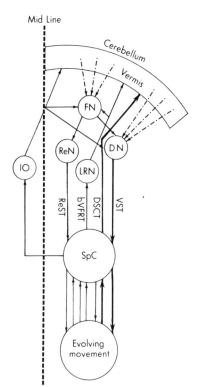

Figure 50. Pathways linking the cerebellar vermis with the spinal centers and so to the evolving movement. bVFRT = bilateral ventral flexor reflex tract; DN = Deiters' nucleus; DSCT = dorsal spino-cerebellar tract; FN = fastigial nucleus; IO = inferior olive; LRN = lateral reticular nucleus; ReN = reticular nucleus; ReST = reticulospinal tract; SpC = spinal centers; VST = vestibulospinal tract. [Eccles, 1973b]

with cerebral command structures. In considering the hierarchy of cerebrocerebellar relationships, Eccles suggested that the command for any limb movement comes from the cerebral cortex, while the cerebellum refines the movement by on-line computations. That this is but one of several possible schemes will emerge later. The physiology of a number of cerebellar pathways has recently been traced by Eccles (1973b). Figure 50 shows the "primitive" vermal system of spino-cerebellar interactions; in Figure 51, the pars intermedia extends the vermal scheme to include cerebral interactions. Cerebral pyramidal axons send collaterals to the nucleus pontis from which emanate the afferents that terminate in mossy fibers on granule cells (cf. Figure 24). There are return pathways to the cerebrum. In the cerebrocerebellar feedback loop in man, it takes about 10 msec for the signal to return, as compared to the signal in the peripheral feedback loop which takes about 100 msec.

The cerebellar pars intermedia (nucleus interpositus) has peripheral feedback and red nucleus output. This scheme (Figure 51) may be viewed as a dynamic control system in which the cerebellar Purkinje

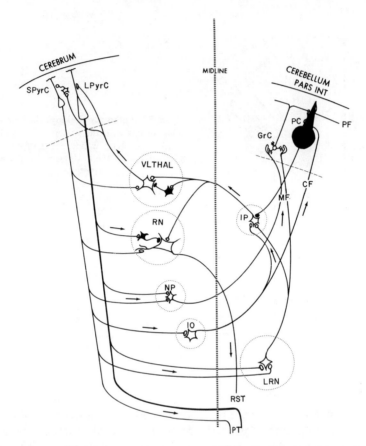

Figure 51. Pathways linking the sensorimotor areas of the cerebrum with the pars intermedia of the cerebellum. CF = climbing fiber; GrC = granule cell; IO = inferior olive; IP = interpositus nucleus; LPyrC = large pyramidal cell; LRN = lateral reticular nucleus; MF = mossy fiber; NP = nuclei pontis; PC = pyramidal cell; PF = pyramidal fiber; PT = pyramidal tract; RN = red nucleus; RST = rubrospinal tract; SPyrC = small pyramidal cell; VLTHAL = ventrolateral thalamus. [Eccles, 1973b]

cells are active all the time unless they are inhibited. As Eccles stated at the Work Session: "We are learning throughout our lifetime, getting a wiser and wiser cerebellum to enable us to make more graceful and efficient movements." As noted above, this view is ahead of the experimental evidence, but it has, in the hands of Marr, led to some interesting network theory. Sabah (1971) has also suggested that there is great redundancy in the cerebellum, which may tie back to the reliability studies of Winograd and Cowan (1963).

In Figure 52, the most highly evolved cerebrocerebellar interactions involving the cerebellar hemispheres are presented. Eccles

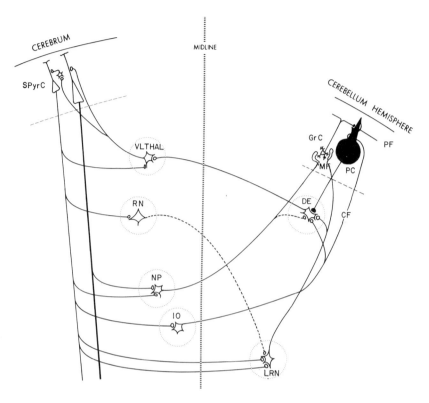

Figure 52. Pathways linking the sensorimotor areas of the cerebrum with the cerebellar hemisphere. CF = climbing fiber; DE = dentate nucleus; GrC = granule cell; IO = inferior olive; LRN = lateral reticular nucleus; MF = mossy fiber; NP = nuclei pontis; PC = Purkinje cell; PF = parallel fiber; RN = red nucleus; SPyrC = small pyramidal cell; VLTHAL = ventrolateral thalamus. [Eccles]

suggested that in this scheme the pontine nuclei (PN), inferior olive (IO), and lateral reticular nuclei (LRN) are all automatically activated by a movement command. Note that granule cells get two types of mossy fiber messages: one from the PN and one from the LRN. Intriguingly, only the LRN mossy fibers send collaterals to the nucleus interpositus, and these are the slower ones—as if the interpositus were designed to receive the direct LRN messages at the same time that it receives the cortically modulated PN messages.

Eccles' views on the relation between cerebrum, cerebellum, and "evolving movements" may be gleaned from his comments on an earlier version of the above figures:

> The cerebellar hemisphere does not receive information directly from the various spinocerebellar pathways [Eccles et al., 1967].

The flow of information from the movement is represented as occurring via the cerebral cortex and is given in the modification of discharge from pyramidal cells. Thus the evolving movement can project sensory information to the cerebellar hemisphere by the following pathway: receptors to spinocerebral pathways to cerebrocerebellar paths through the pontine nuclei and the principal olive. The integration of the presumed diverse subsets of corticocerebellar information will occur in the evolving movement . . . but of course it will also occur in the immense and complex association paths in the cerebral hemispheres. Figure 7B [Figure 7B refers to Eccles' original Figure 51] shows diagrammatically the more complex circuitry that is postulated to operate in movement control by the intermediate zone of the anterior lobe in the cerebellum. It will be seen that there are three locations at which integration can occur in the cerebral and cerebellar contributions to the control of movement: in the cerebral cortex with expression in the pyramidal cell discharge; in the cerebellar cortex with expression in the Purkinje cell discharge; and in the spinal cord where the motoneuronal discharge finds expression in the evolving movement.

There are three components of this hypothesis of the operative circuits by which the cerebellum controls movement. Firstly, there is the input into a multitude of independent integrating areas of the cerebellar cortex of very diverse subsets of information from the receptors activated by the movement and by the cortical controlling centers [Eccles et al., 1968a,b]. Secondly, the piecemeal integration so effected is transmitted in the cerebellar efferents both to the spinal cord and to the cerebral cortex and is unified provisionally in the neuronal mechanisms of the cerebral cortex and spinal cord, but finally in the changes produced in the evolving movement. Thirdly, the changes in the evolving movement are fed back by receptor organ discharges to the cerebellum and to the cerebral cortex, so completing the operational circuits, which are shown in the several diagrams. It is an essential part of the hypothesis that there is a continual feedback of information to the cerebellar integrating mechanisms. All integrations there are piecemeal and provisional. The coherence and smoothness of movements are achieved by the circuits that are continuously in operation not only during a movement but in all sequences of movement [Eccles, 1967].

More recent studies have stressed the distinction between slow and fast fibers and their role in cerebellar organization. This is best summarized in the diagram of a spatiotemporal plot of impulse

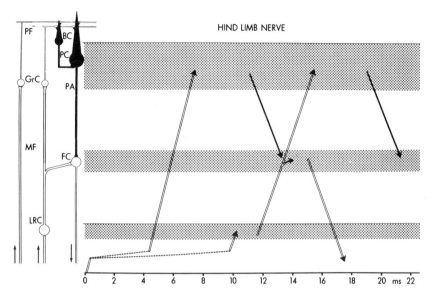

Figure 53. Spatiotemporal plot of impulse transmission to and from the cerebellum for responses evoked by stimulation of a hindlimb nerve. The horizontal bands symbolize the areas of neurons and synapses, from below upwards the lateral reticular cells (LRC), the fastigial cells (FC), and the cerebellar cortex, as illustrated in the diagram at the left. BC = basket cell; GrC = granule cell; MF = mossy fiber; PA = Purkinje axon; PC = Purkinje cell; PF = parallel fiber. [Eccles, 1973a]

transmission through the cerebellum (Figure 53), which according to Eccles (1973a) is constructed in order to:

> ... display the times of impulse discharges and ... propagations [along] the various pathways illustrated to the left [with standard nomenclature. Note that the nuclear areas are shown by dotted zones in the main diagram, and that impulse transmission is demonstrated by the sloped lines, with the horizontal scale giving time in milliseconds from the stimulus to a hindlimb nerve.] Nerve stimulation at zero time results in a fast mossy fibre volley via the dorsal spino-cerebellar tract that reaches the cerebellar cortex in about 7 msec. It is shown with an intercept by ... [a broken line] that signifies the long traject up [the] peripheral nerve and spinal cord. The slower mossy fibre pathway via the bVFR tract is shown also with an intercept, finally reaching the lateral reticular nucleus at about 10 msec latency and evoking a discharge that propagates up to the cerebellum ... [with] a collateral to the fastigial nucleus. . . . this collateral evokes from the fastigial cell a discharge after a delay of a millisecond or so, that is plotted as the downward sloping

arrow. . . . Meanwhile the fast mossy fibre input to the cerebellum will have produced a Purkyně* cell discharge [back] to the fastigial nucleus, as shown by the solid downward sloping arrow. The plotted times of discharge correspond with the average values for a large number of experiments and reveal that the Purkyně cell discharge arrives at the fastigial nucleus at approximate simultaneity with [the impulse resulting from] the lateral reticular discharge. This is the optimal timing for the [effective] interaction of these two opposed synaptic actions.

Eccles (1969b) added that the findings of Merton and his co-workers (1967) on tremor can be accounted for by feedback via the external loop of Figure 52. Greene (1972) has reviewed the Russian work (Aizerman and Andreeva, 1968a,b; Chernov, 1968, Andreeva et al., 1969; Aizerman and Gurfinkel, 1970), which shows that, when one is holding the arm in a particular position, opposing muscles alternately pull the arm one way and then the other way, producing a tremor of about 10 cycles per sec. Greene commented that this form of control by rapid alternations of opposing influences has a well-known linearizing effect upon any system to which it is applied, thus allowing graded control ("proportional control") to be exerted by highly nonlinear and discontinuous systems, such as relays (MacColl, 1945, Loeb, 1952; Cosgriff, 1958; Graham and McRuer, 1961). For example, a model airplane, remotely controlled by relays, can be steered continously by rapidly moving the rudder left and right in time-biased alternation. In general, a rapidly fluctuating signal, sometimes called a "dither," may be added to a slowly varying control signal in order to remove a threshold, or to "unstick" friction, or to make a system element behave more like an ideal linear element. For example, if a relay is rapidly turned on and off by an alternating current, causing the controlled output voltage to alternate between positive and negative constants of equal magnitude, then the average voltage in the controlled output and, hence, the average torque on the shaft of a controlled motor, is proportional to the difference between the time the relay is on and the time the relay is off. This difference is nearly proportional to a small, slowly varying bias signal added to the alternating current.

In the nervous system, this linearization may further simplify the task of control by making different nonlinearities look similar to the controller, which thereby might be enabled to employ a uniform method for producing similar movement patterns, using different muscle groups having different nonlinear characteristics.

*Eccles now prefers to use the original Czech spelling, as did Purkyně himself, to the form Purkinje, which is standard in the literature and is used elsewhere in this *Bulletin*.

Cerebellar Projections

While the structure of the cerebellar cortex is similar through-out its entirety, there is considerable functional differentiation owing to various areas having different input and output connections. Figure 54 shows the spinal projection areas as demonstrated by Snider (1952). The double representation in the anterior and the posterior lobes, respectively (another example of multiple topographic represen-tations discussed in Chapter II), is largely obtained by the branching of climbing and mossy fibers to innervate corresponding areas in the two regions (Cooke et al., 1971; Armstrong et al., 1973a,b,c).

The spinal input to the cerebellar cortex is carried by about twenty different paths. Only two mossy fiber paths, the cuneocere-bellar tract (for the forelimb) and the dorsal spinocerebellar tract (for the hindlimb), carry information directly related to peripheral events. All other climbing and mossy fiber paths have an organization that suggests that they serve as internal feedback paths that monitor the activity in lower motor centers (see Figure 55 and the discussion in

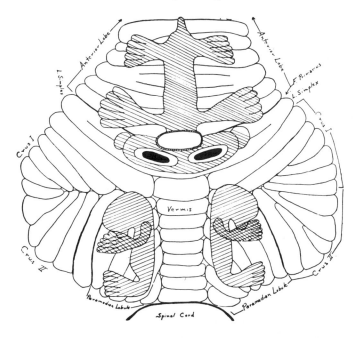

Figure 54. Outline drawing of the cerebellum showing the tactile areas in schematized form. The anterior area encompasses the lobulus simplex and anterior lobe and is an ipsilateral projection. The posterior area is located primarily in the paramedian lobules bilaterally but may extend into crus I and II and medially into pyramis. Note body plan in each tactile area; it is less definite in contralateral paramedian lobule than in other areas. [Snider, 1952]

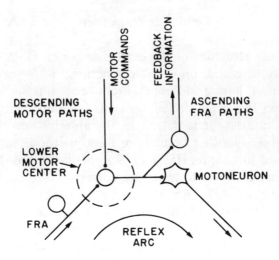

Figure 55. Suggested function of ascending paths from the flexor reflex afferents (FRA). It is assumed that these paths monitor activity in lower motor centers whose pools of interneurons are both reflex arcs and links in descending motor paths. [Oscarsson, 1971]

Evarts et al., 1971, pp. 100-101). This hypothesis is strongly supported by recent studies on the ventral spinocerebellar tract. Neurons of this tract often receive only a weak, direct input from primary afferents but are strongly influenced by spinal interneurons that mediate segmental reflexes and descending motor commands (Lundberg, 1971; Lindström, 1973). Furthermore, the rhythmic activity in ventral spinocerebellar tract neurons that can be recorded during stepping in mesencephalic cats persists after deafferentation (Arshavsky et al., 1972).

Topography of the Spinal Projection

The principles of the topography of the spinal projection to the cerebellar cortex were presented at the Work Session by Larson, using the forelimb area in the pars intermedia of the anterior lobe as a model. The simplified diagram in Figure 56 shows that the climbing fiber input is organized in four narrow sagittal zones, c_1, c_2, c_3, and d (cf. Oscarsson, 1973). It is possible that these zones correspond to the four zones identified by Voogd (1969) using anatomical techniques. The climbing fiber zones run continuously throughout superficial and deep parts of the folia, oriented perpendicular to the long axis of the folia.* Note that Figure 56 illustrates only a small part of the projection area: two adjacent folia and the interposed sulcus that are shown unfolded.

*C. -F. Ekerot and B. Larson, manuscript in preparation.

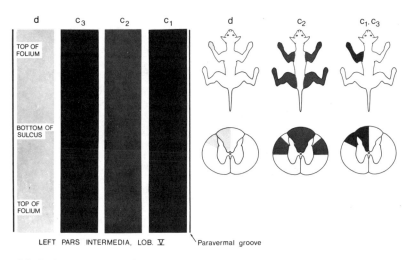

Figure 56. Projection of spinal climbing fiber paths to the forelimb area in the pars intermedia of the anterior lobe. Only two adjacent folia and the interposed sulcus are shown unfolded. The receptive fields of each zone (c_1, c_2, c_3, and d) and the location of the paths in the cervical cord are shown at the right. See the text for details. [Larson]

The c_1 and c_3 zones receive a similar climbing fiber input from the ipsilateral forelimb. The projection to these zones via the dorsal funiculus represents the most direct path from the forelimb to the pars intermedia. In the c_3 zone this projection has been shown to have a crude somatotopical organization (Ekerot and Larson, 1973). Each part of the forelimb is represented along the entire zone. The paw is represented in the middle of the zone and the more proximal portions of the limb are represented in its medial and lateral parts.

The kind of information that is carried by the climbing fiber systems is uncertain. In preparations with only one spinal path intact, natural stimulation is usually rather ineffective although electrical stimulation of cutaneous and high-threshold muscle afferents is very effective (Oscarsson, 1973). Furthermore, the olivary and presumably the preolivary relays are controlled by higher centers. Oscarsson has therefore suggested that the climbing fiber paths carry information about the activity in lower motor centers rather than about peripheral events. On the other hand, it has recently been demonstrated that climbing fiber responses can be evoked by light mechanical stimuli applied to the skin in small receptive fields (Eccles et al., 1972d,e; Leicht et al., 1973). It is, of course, still possible that these responses signal a specific change in the activity of lower motor centers caused by the peripheral input.

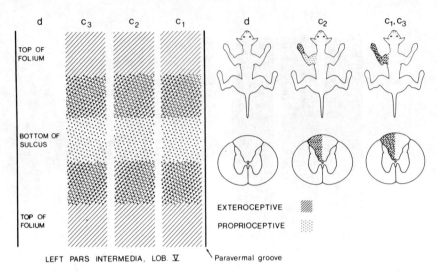

Figure 57. Projection of the cuneocerebellar tract to the same region of the cerebellar cortex as shown in Figure 56. See the text for details. [Larson]

Figure 57 shows the main features of the cuneocerebellar projection to the same cortical area as shown in Figure 56. As discussed above, this tract terminates as mossy fibers and conveys information directly related to peripheral events. This input is arranged in sagittal zones that overlap the climbing fiber zones, c_1, c_2, and c_3 (Ekerot and Larson, 1973), but with the distinctive difference that the projection from exteroceptors and proprioceptors is discontinuous according to the foliation of the cerebellar cortex (Ekerot and Larson, 1972). While the exteroceptive mossy fiber input favors the top of the folia, the proprioceptive input (from group I muscle afferents) is confined to the depth of the sulci (also shown in sagittal section in Figure 58). Thus, foliation is not just a way of fitting a large cortical sheet into the skull; it also represents a functional subdivision of the cerebellar cortex in alternating transverse bands receiving mossy fiber inputs from extero-ceptors and proprioceptors, respectively. It is interesting that in degeneration studies other mossy fiber systems have also been shown to terminate according to the foliation (Voogd, 1967).

The mossy fiber zones in Figure 57 were revealed by recording the synaptic field potentials evoked in the granular layer. In the molecular layer the narrow gaps between neighboring zones would be "blurred" owing to the spread of activity via the parallel fibers. This is the case for both the proprioceptive input and the exteroceptive input from the paw that project to all the zones, i.e., c_1, c_2, and c_3. However,

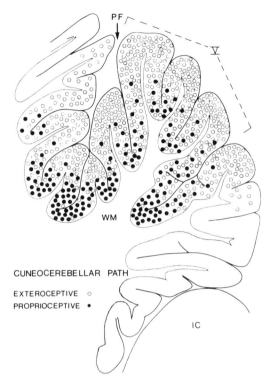

Figure 58. Projection of the cuneocerebellar tract. Sagittal section through the pars intermedia of the anterior lobe. IC = inferior colliculus; PF = primary fissure; WM = white matter. [Larson]

the zonal organization can be recognized in the molecular layer for the exteroceptive input from more proximal parts of the forelimb that project only to the c_1 and c_3 zones. In this case the parallel fiber activity does not completely bridge the c_2 and d zones.*

The sagittal climbing fiber zones and the transverse mossy fiber bands subdivide the cerebellar cortex into an orthogonal lattice with many different .combinations of climbing and mossy fiber inputs (imagine the projection areas in Figures 56 and 57 superimposed and continuing over several folia). In some regions, at the top of the folia in the c_1 and c_3 zones, there is a clear parallelism between the climbing and mossy fiber inputs that can be elicited by stimulation of skin nerves (Eccles et al., 1972e; Ekerot and Larson, 1973). In the deep parts of these zones, however, the same climbing fiber input is combined with a proprioceptive mossy fiber input. Other combinations occur in the c_2 and d zones.

*C. -F. Ekerot and B. Larson, unpublished observations.

The anatomical basis of this complex system of projections in the cerebellum has been clarified by the elegant studies of Voogd (1969). He showed that the termination of afferent systems in a series of parallel (concentric) sagittal strips of the cerebellar cortex is not due primarily and exclusively to the differential projections of various afferent systems but, rather, to certain systematic changes in myelo-architectonics, i.e., regions of accumulations of fibers of fine caliber in the medullary laminas (the so-called "raphes" of Voogd, 1964) arranged at roughly equal distances from each other and from the midline. These raphes subdivide the median lobe (vermis proper) into a compartment, or zone a, adjacent to the midline and zone b laterally; the intermediate lobe can be subdivided in mediolateral sequence into compartments or zones, c_1, c_2, c_3, and d, already mentioned in the preceding paragraphs in connection with the projection of the forelimb to lobe V of the cerebellum.

Lesions of the spino- and cuneocerebellar pathways result in a discontinuous distribution of terminal degeneration within the frontal plane, showing maxima of degeneration both in the white laminas and in the granular layer generally in or close to the border of the several zones. The olivocerebellar projections show the same compartmental-ization into parallel sagittal zones, as might be expected from the physiological observations of Oscarsson and Uddenberg (1964), how-ever, the difference is that the degeneration maxima tend sometimes to match up with the zone rather than with its borders.

The termination of mossy afferents in relatively narrow, sagittally oriented zones of the cerebellar cortex automatically raises the question of whether parallel fiber activity would blur the borders between neighboring zones, and, if so, how far it would do so. Braitenberg suggested that the degree of overlap between the parallel fiber populations arising from neighboring compartments might be just the essential part of the computation. According to Larson, the longitudinal zones of mossy fiber input from a similar source are 0.5 to 1 mm in width in the cat. He has shown that, although the gap between c_1 and c_3 for proximal exteroceptive input might be narrowed by the parallel fibers, it would not be closed entirely. As Szentágothai pointed out, the anatomical data of Voogd and the physiological observations of Larson agree with the recent statistical finding of 2 mm as the length of parallel fibers in the cat, as reported by Palkovits and his colleagues (1971c). In the adult cat, six sagittal zones (or strips) are contained in the anterior lobe, which is 7-mm wide from the midline to its lateral border. Hence, slightly above 1 mm is available, on the average, for each zone. Consequently, the parallel fibers arising from cells at the border between two zones (close to the raphes of Voogd) would traverse both neighboring zones almost completely, while the parallel fibers arising from granule cells situated in the centers of one zone would invade the two adjacent zones close to halfway. For purely anatomical reasons, one would thus expect that the gaps between neighboring sagittal zones would be completely bridged by parallel fibers of 2-mm length. However, there should be no overlapping of parallel fibers from alternate zones, e.g., c_1 and c_3. This is interesting from the viewpoint that there is virtually no interaction by parallel fibers between zones c_1 and c_3, which have the same exteroceptor mossy and climbing fiber input from the upper limb (see Figures 56 and 57).

The efferent corticonuclear projection is also based on the sagittal zone principle (Jansen and Brodal, 1940, 1942). Accordingly, the cerebellar cortex of the rabbit is divided into four longitudinal zones (in mediolateral sequence): a projecting to the fastigial nucleus, b projecting to the lateral vestibular nucleus, c projecting to the interpositus nucleus, and d projecting to the lateral nucleus.

Numerical Input-Output Relations

Another aspect of the cerebellar projections that was discussed during the Work Session and deserves more detailed scrutiny is the input-output relations. The numerical relations of afferent to efferent fibers according to Van der Loos and Ramón-Moliner are grossly disproportionate in the cerebellum as compared to the cerebrum. If one regards as cerebellar output that which originates in the deep cerebellar nuclei, then the cerebellum has obviously a small output compared to its massive input. In the forebrain (cortex plus thalamus) the situation is reversed: the number of ascending afferent fibers to the thalamus is probably less than that of the fibers present in the cerebral peduncle. On closer inspection, however, certain other qualifications become necessary. The number of afferent fibers compared to the number of Purkinje cells is by no means excessive. If the inferior olive is considered as the sole source of climbing fibers (which is by no means certain), then the original number of these afferents makes up only 10% of the slightly above 10^6 Purkinje cells in the cat.* The 4:1 ratio of mossy fibers to Purkinje cells, found by Palkovits and his co-workers

---

*Since the ratio of climbing fiber branches to Purkinje cells is undoubtedly close to 1:1 in the cerebellar cortex, it would be expected that the average original climbing fiber must branch into ten fibers during its course in the white matter.

(1972) for smaller, well-isolated folia, cannot be extended to the entire cerebellum since mossy afferents are known to branch in the white matter below the base of the folia (see Figure 41 in Ramón y Cajal, 1911). If one assumes a single branching of the average mossy afferent for two folia, then the total number of mossy afferents (main stems) in the cat cerebellum would be expected to be around 2.4×10^6. Palkovits and his co-workers (1972) consider this estimate too high and suggest a more abundant branching of the mossy afferents. Hence, the numerical input-output ratio for the cerebellar cortex itself could not possibly be much higher than 2:1 and is probably less. The situation changes radically when considering the number of nuclear efferents. Estimates on the degree of convergence from Purkinje cells to nuclear neurons run between 20 and 50.* The direct corticovestibular efferents can change this ratio only insignificantly. Thus, the total input-output fiber ratio of the cerebellum would be around 50-60:1, which is indeed excessive.

Unfortunately, no reliable data on the cerebrum are available; such data would depend on what would be considered the output. The number of projective elements of the cerebral cortex (probably the vast majority of the pyramidal cells) is grossly larger than that of the afferents. A more realistic input-output ratio can be obtained by comparing the total number of fibers in the base of the cerebral peduncles (output) with the number of ascending fibers in the anterior segment of the midbrain plus the number of optic and afferent olfactory tract fibers. It is debatable, though, whether such numbers would be meaningful at all in the cerebrum with its immense internal connectivity.

The convergence of numerous Purkinje cell axons upon each projective nuclear neuron of the cerebellum is of great significance and received much attention from Eccles (1971). Since, in addition to convergence, there is also some divergence in the Purkinje cell-nuclear cell relay (see Figure 125 in Eccles et al., 1967), the functional circumstances of the transfer become rather complicated (Eccles, 1971). Using the tools of information theory to discover how the nuclear neurons might be used to forward information about the

---

*A recent unpublished study by Palkovits and his co-workers in the 1st Anatomy Department of Semmelweis University Medical School in Budapest gives the crude Purkinje cell to nuclear cell ratio as 27:1, provided that all nuclear cells are projective neurons (this latter assumption is unconfirmed and is still under study).

functional states of partially overlapping sets of Purkinje cells, from which nuclear neurons receive their convergent inputs, could be a rewarding study. What kind of neural coding would be needed to separate the information arising from various subsets corresponding to various overlaps? If there is only convergence, each nuclear cell would represent a definite set of Purkinje cells. However, if there is additional divergence, the representation of any Purkinje cell by the nuclear neurons would become nonunique. In this case, the nervous system would presumably take information as coded in terms of configurations of activity of Purkinje cells.

Features of the Cerebellar Relay Systems

Unusual common features of the cerebellar relay systems—both the afferent and efferent—are: (1) the separation of the immediate pre- and (some) postcerebellar nuclei from the general neuropil, and/or (2) the tendency towards the separation of the dendritic arborization spaces of individual cells. These features are discussed in detail in the following paragraphs:

1. The separation of the dendritic and axonal arborizations from the surrounding neuropil is obvious and well known from the early classic studies of Clarke's column (see Figure 145 in Ramón y Cajal, 1909). Such nuclei have been labeled "noyaux fermés" (Mannen, 1960), and, as stressed by Szentágothai and Albert (1955), this structural arrangement is suggestive of the functional separation of the nucleus and its neuropil from the general neuropil of the cord. The same tendency is apparent in the lateral reticular nucleus; however, it tends to decrease or almost disappear in the primates. Conversely, the tendency is reversed in the inferior olive where the separation of the neuropil becomes really apparent in the primates, particularly in man. The anatomical situation of the postcerebellar nuclei is such that there is no surrounding neuropil with which the neuropil of the nuclei could merge.

2. The establishment of individual dendritic arborization spaces and private neuropil compartments is a general tendency both phylogenetically and ontogenetically in the inferior olive. This reaches its maximum in the human where we can almost directly visualize the complete transformation of the randomly radiating dendritic tree of the fetus into the idiodendritic tree (see Chapter III) of the olive cells

having all recurring branches at the age of 2 months. The same process occurs in the dentate nucleus of primates (see Figure 125 in Eccles et al., 1967). The result, in terms of connectivity, is that each of the cells in these nuclei establishes a private synaptic neuropil, and transmission to each of them can be a highly individual matter, certainly more so than one might suppose in nuclei where both dendrites and axonal arborizations are intricately interwoven. Recently, Llinás and his collaborators (1973) reported their findings on electrical coupling between inferior olivary cells of the cat with corresponding "tight junctions" between dendrites. Their data indicate that local assemblies of olivary cells might be functionally generated. This implies that, in nuclei having noninterpenetrating dendritic arborizations (idiodendritic cell types), dendritic interactions are confined to cells in each other's immediate neighborhood, whereas in interpenetrating dendritic arrangements such interactions might extend to larger groups of nerve cells.

The elegant concept of Ramón-Moliner and Nauta (1966) on the systematics of dendritic arborization and the general thoughts added in the above section on "Randomness Versus Specificity of Structure" (Chapter III) are certainly applicable to the study of the afferent and efferent connections of the cerebellum. The cells in almost all the specific precerebellar nuclei (Ramón-Moliner, 1968) are either allodendritic (Clarke's column, external cuneate nucleus, pontine nuclei) or idiodendritic (inferior olive), with the consequences already discussed (Figure 59). Therefore, perhaps the following interpretation is not too farfetched: the cerebellar system as a whole, including most of its afferent and efferent connections, exhibits a high degree of structural differentiation (and specialization) with the net result that everything seems to be determined to the fullest extent by (1) the geometry of arborizations, (2) the positions (or arrangements) of cells and arborizations in space, and (3) the numerical and topological features (parameters) of cells and branchings. Of course, one might argue that, within the less regular, denser entanglements in other central organs, the same degree, or more, of strictly determined wiring might prevail. No matter what is the case, we would have to ask: "What might be the meaning of such unusual regularity and structural refinement that appears very early in vertebrate phylogeny (as, for example, in the shape and arrangement of the Purkinje cells) and then is so emphatically maintained and further developed and extended to the high degree found in man?"

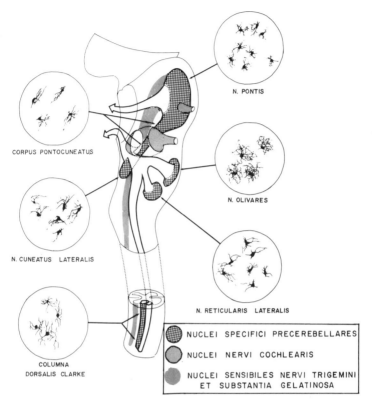

Figure 59. Most specific precerebellar nuclei are characterized by the presence of allodendritic and even idiodendritic neurons, with a more or less marked tendency to dendritic waviness. [Ramón-Moliner]

Synergies and Cerebellar Function

The skeletomuscular system presents an enormous number of physical degrees of freedom to its controller. Yet the works of Bernstein, Gelfand, Tsetlin, and Greene (reviewed in Chapter II) suggest that this rich apparatus is directed with rather simple executive commands, which are implemented via the so-called low-level "function generators" between the executive and the periphery that constrain large subsets of the free variables.

The Russian Perspective

In the present section, we shall see how the Bernstein (1967; Gelfand et al., 1971) control paradigm has provided the framework within which Boylls (1975) has developed a theory of cerebellar functioning for the mesencephalic cat. Since the absence of forebrain "reduces" the cerebellum functionally to its spinal and vestibular divisions, the emphasis of the theory is on the anterior lobe. In the mesencephalic (or thalamic) locomoting cat, the delivery of constant stimulation to a midbrain "locomotory region" awakens an elaborate neuronal assembly, yielding well-coordinated locomotion upon a treadmill; the stimulus intensity appears only to specify the energy output of the performance (Shik et al., 1966).

What are the subordinate function generators translating a locomotory region command into action? It is now known that the cat spinal cord contains a sketchy algorithm for progression (Forssberg and Grillner, 1973). That program is, in turn, probably selected by reticular centers (Grillner and Shik, 1973) receiving excitation from the locomotory region through unknown channels (Orlovskii, 1970a). Inflow from the cerebellum, however, is essential to the artful execution of an otherwise "ataxic" locomotory pattern (Orlovskii, 1970b), for it modulates the synergic relations of muscle groups, i.e., the constraints or linkages that convert them into a few economically controlled sets.

According to Boylls, cerebellar influences on synergic construction in mesencephalic locomotion are expressed in spatiotemporal neuronal activity patterns created in the motor "output nuclei" of the brainstem, namely, the red and Deiters' nuclei and certain reticular centers; indeed, modulation of cerebellar target nuclei during locomotion ceases with cerebellar ablation (Orlovskii, 1970b, 1972a,b). Boylls confines his theorizing to red and Deiters' nuclei, each well known to possess a topographic organization relative to the musculature influenced. The red nucleus preferentially excites functional flexors, while Deiters' nucleus has somewhat complementary influences upon extensors (Pompeiano, 1967). The interpositus and fastigial cerebellar nuclei that excite red and Deiters' nuclei, respectively, exhibit corresponding topographies and muscular affinities. For example, a particular synergic utilization of hindlimb flexors and extensors must possess a corresponding "encoding" in unique spatiotemporal activity patterns within the interpositus and fastigial nuclei. This suggests that any cerebellar influence on such a synergy is obtained by creating these activity encodings under supervision of the cerebellar cortex and its afferents, certain cerebellar reticular nuclei, and the astonishing neural connectivity geometries relating these components.

Boylls's Synergy Controller Model

The cerebellar "computer" of the resultant model is diagrammed in Figure 60. Keep in mind that its purpose is to create synergically meaningful excitation profiles on a cerebellar nucleus, which are subsequently transmitted via an "output nucleus" to spinal levels. The principal instrument of this pattern sculpting is, of course, spatiotemporally significant inhibition from the cerebellar cortex; but this, in turn, results from activity on climbing fibers of the inferior olive and on both "slow" and "fast" mossy fiber paths (Figure 53).*

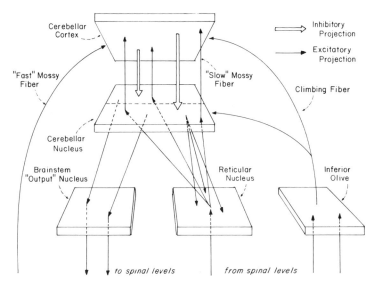

Figure 60. Components of cerebellar related circuitry and their interconnections, as conceived in Boylls's theory of cerebellar function in mesencephalic locomotion. [Arbib et al., 1974]

A crucial addition to this classic story is the inclusion in the model of so-called "reverberatory" or positive-feedback connections between the cerebellar nuclei and particular reticular nuclei. Such loop activity must also reach the cerebellar cortex on slow mossy fibers, thereby creating a negative-feedback check on an otherwise unstable situation. Figure 61 depicts the reverberatory connection between a typical cerebellar (interpositus) and cerebellum-related reticular nucleus (reticularis tegmenti pontis). Anatomically, the work of Brodal and his

---

*Later developments of such models will have to incorporate the inhibitory interneurons of the cerebellar cortex. This story will be complicated by the rich connections of climbing fibers to the interneurons, which are only now receiving careful experimental study.

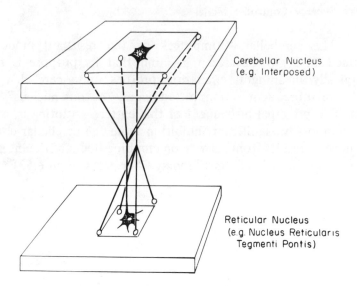

Figure 61. Anatomical template scheme of reticulocerebellar reverberatory loop (positive feedback) connectivity. [Arbib et al., 1974]

colleagues (Brodal and Szikla, 1972; Brodal et al., 1972) suggests that the cerebellofugal projection may display rather more topographic precision than does the reverberatory return in the projection between the interpositus and the nucleus reticularis tegmenti pontis. The geometry of the projection is indicated in template fashion (Figure 61) for one typical neuron of each nucleus. Similarly, Tsukahara (1972) has provided physiological data, first, on the aggregate behavior of this loop, showing that it does support reverberatory activity in the absence of cerebellar cortical inhibiton and, secondly, on the neurons of each nucleus, for instance, the time course of the excitatory postsynaptic potential. Simulation of this loop region, then, merely involves the use of two populations of model neurons interconnected in space by the templates shown in Figure 61. Mathematically, this becomes a system of coupled, nonlinear differential equations over space and time, whose activity is then observed by using computer graphics. Similar equations are generated by the other structures of Figure 60.

In Figure 62 the cerebellopetal fibers of the reticular nucleus are shown continuing to the cerebellar cortex as slow mossy fibers after having made nuclear collateral synapses. This initial caricature of the cortex embodies the frog-like "basic cerebellar circuit" of Llinás (1970), wherein only granule and Purkinje cells and parallel, mossy, and climbing fibers are recognized, along with the related geometry (certain

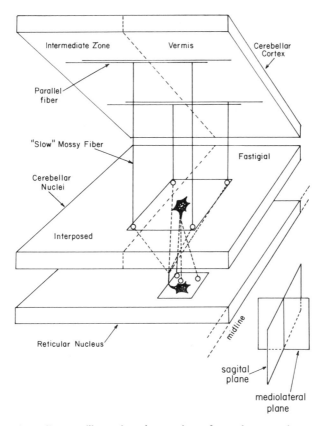

Figure 62. Template diagram illustrating the routing of reverberatory loop activity to a simplified cerebellar cortex via a subset of slow mossy fibers. Not shown are the granular and Purkinje layers, nor the actual spatial geometry of mossy fibers as they arrive at the cortex. Boylls treats the branching of the mossy fibers as if they were lying mostly in a sagittal plane but with a substantial mediolateral excursion (see the text). [Arbib et al., 1974]

of these elements are omitted from Figure 62 for clarity). This proved qualitatively sufficient to establish the observations below. In later work, however, a refined rendition of granular layer processing is created (employing an experimentally testable, motoneuron-like recruitment hypothesis that has phylogenetic basis), along with a mathematical representation of temporal aspects of cortical interneuronal effects (Murphy et al., 1973b).

The addition of sagittal-mediolateral coordinate planes should also be noted in Figure 62. These are set up relative to the cortex (i.e., with parallel fibers coursing mediolaterally, etc.) and serve to peg homologous nuclear regions. The geometric distributions of climbing and mossy fibers, and of the cerebellar corticonuclear projection, are also visualized in the coordinate scheme and modeled accordingly. Boylls contends that, for the cat anterior lobe, there is considerable evidence that all routes to and from the cortex are basically sagittally oriented, with varying amounts of mediolateral spread (see also Szentágothai above). He is thus in general agreement with Voogd (1969) who reported that the cerebellum shows a sagittal compartmentalization "bridged" by parallel fibers. (For more recent work related to this problem, see Murphy et al., 1973a; Armstrong et al., 1973a,b.)

Only a few of the more interesting results of the computer simulation of this cerebellum model can be given here. Climbing fiber inputs produce an initial collateral activation of the cerebellar nuclei followed by a brief, strong burst of Purkinje cell activity prior to the so-called "inactivation response" of Granit and Phillips (1956). The last is a silencing of the Purkinje cell for a highly variable length of time, depending on the preparation employed (see, for instance, Murphy and Sabah, 1970; Murphy et al., 1973b); etiology of the inactivation continues to be in dispute. Boylls's simulation employs a brief, 16-msec inactivation following a very strong Purkinje burst, with sagittal zone distribution of the affected cells—supposedly as would be produced by activation of a small region of the inferior olive (Armstrong et al., 1973a). The cerebellar nuclear aftermath of this is shown in Figure 63. Above the nucleus, a rolling surface indicates by its height the degree of excitation of nuclear cells. The central, sagittal "hill" is located at the homologue of the activated cortical strip and is flanked by two depressed regions. This hill was created when the Purkinje inactivation response released underlying nuclear cells from cortical inhibition. At the same time, however, the rebounding nuclear activity was greatly amplified through the reticulonuclear reverberation (positive feedback), which not only serves to maintain the hill but is also transmitted back to the cortex; there, it spreads mediolaterally along parallel fibers, activating more Purkinje cells and thus leading to simple lateral inhibition of the nuclear areas adjacent to the hill. The persistence of this spatial excitation configuration is partially regulated by the ratio of positive to negative feedback gain in the system. In the simulation, the pattern (which otherwise fades) is "refreshed" by climbing fiber input about every 100 msec, in keeping with the approximate firing periodicities of the olivary cell ensemble (Bell and Kawasaki, 1972).

What do such patterns mean? Boylls looks initially at the synergic interpretation, i.e., at the encoding implied by the pattern of Figure 63. Regardless of specific cerebellar nuclear topography, if this

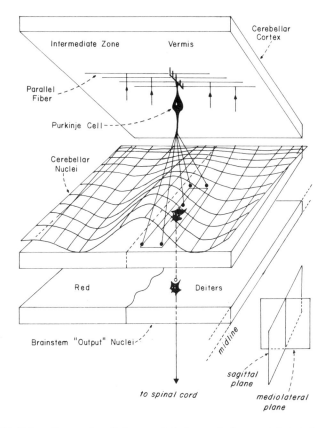

Figure 63. Spatial pattern of activity created in cerebellar nuclei (relative to cortical coordinates) by climbing fiber action along one sagittal strip in Boylls's computer simulation (height of the functional surface indicates magnitude of excitation at each locus). The active climbing fiber strip was located in the cortex above the central hill of excitation shown. This hill and the depressed valleys flanking it persist for a considerable time beyond the initiating climbing fiber bursts (for mechanisms of this phenomenon, see the text). Such patterns are transmitted to various brainstem motor nuclei and are topographically interpretable as "programs" for cerebellar synergic modulation. [Arbib et al., 1974]

pattern directly modulates the musculature, those muscles represented within the sagittal hill of excitation would tend to co-contract—they would be agonists of a synergy (to employ Boylls's terms). Contrariwise, muscles within the adjacent "valleys" would simultaneously co-relax as synergic antagonists. Translating this into cerebellar cortical coordinates, one concludes that, along any sagittal climbing fiber zone of the cortex, certain synergic agonists can be recruited by climbing fiber action, whereas along the mediolateral dimension their antagonists are suppressed on either side of the zone. Interpreting the data of the earlier section, we may suggest that Voogd (1969) and Oscarsson (1969) have mapped out the cortex in a way that allows some specification of the actual synergic linkages wrought in each region of the cortex. Voogd's delimiting of the sagittal cerebellar corticonuclear projection describes the cortex in its flexor-extensor influence (since the muscular effects from the cerebellar nuclei are known). Oscarsson's maps of climbing fiber zones divide the same cortex into hindlimb and forelimb regions. Consequently, applying the above synergic formula to each cortical sector can define the flexor-extensor, hindlimb-forelimb synergic modulation possible there. Behavioral tests of these predictions, by using appropriate lesions, can now follow. Divisions of the inferior olive can similarly be assigned synergic (specifically, agonist recruitment) significance. How do cerebellar nuclear activation patterns arrive at the muscles? Is it that they are created by climbing fiber activation just prior to each particular use of some synergy? This need not be so. Orlovsky (1972b) has demonstrated that stimulation of either red or Deiters' nucleus is effective in augmenting contraction of the related musculature *only when that musculature is being actively employed.* It is as though there were a "spinal switch" routing in cerebellar influences only at proper times. Thus, a nuclear activation pattern for some synergy could be built up gradually through climbing fiber activation, and then remain "resident," refreshed at intervals as in Boylls's model. Indeed, red and Deiters' nuclei do show maintained activity even when their related muscles are silent during locomotion (Orlovsky, 1972a,b). The hypothesis awaits direct test, however. It is worth noting that the switching notion is at least as old as Magnus' classic demonstration of "die Umkehr" (Sherrington, 1910), recently reexamined and supported by Grillner;* it is also suggested in work such as that of Kots and Syrovegin (1966). Note also that climbing fiber firing needs to have little temporal correlation with ongoing muscular performance, as was shown by Thach (1968). Yet olivary disruption can result in the abolition of the cerebellar, synergic coordination function, as was found by Murphy and O'Leary (1971).

While the climbing fibers specify the relational nature of synergies in the model, i.e., the specific muscle groups involved and the signs of their covariances, various mossy fiber inputs yield the synergic "metrics": on deployment of each synergy, mossy fibers determine how much contraction to employ. A metric specification is thus not

---

*S. Grillner, personal communication to C. C. Boylls.

unlike that of the "local sign" of a spinal reflex whose muscular relations are fixed (as in the nociceptive flexion reflex (Sherrington, 1910)). Boylls has examined the effects of various types of mossy perturbations on the nuclear synergic patterns set up by climbing fibers. Perturbations delivered at one locus flow through the circuitry smoothly to many other loci over time, thereby achieving, perhaps, the plastic cohesiveness observed in synergies under normal cerebellar control. Finally, relative to decerebrate locomotion, he deduces that major spinocerebellar paths are principally regulating extensor (i.e., support phase) activity. It is known that extension, indeed, provides the significant control variables in quadruped locomotion; flexion (transfer) phases over many velocities are highly standardized (Arshavskii et al., 1965).

Thus, in Greene's terms (see Chapter II), the climbing fibers of Boylls's model establish the synergic "function generation" properties of cerebellar modulation, while the mossy fibers tune these generators. Generator output is switched into the musculature only at particular times, although the generator itself runs continuously, ever updated by feedback and prepared for instant action. The output of each possible generator configuration represents a synergic program. While the term synergy has not been explicitly defined here, it is evident that the traditional Sherringtonian usage is too restrictive to capture the concepts described above. Synergies are features of movement in the same sense that lines or spatial frequencies are considered features of vision. One now awaits a redefinition of synergies to revitalize motor system research along the behavioral lines of investigation successfully used in the visual system.

ABBREVIATIONS

AF	asymmetric membrane contact, flattened vesicle
AOT	accessory optic tract
BC	basket cell
CF	climbing fiber
CFr	climbing fiber response
CN	cerebellar nuclei
CNS	central nervous system
FRA	flexor reflex afferents
GrC	granule cell
IO	inferior olive
LGB	lateral geniculate body
LGN	lateral geniculate nucleus
LRN	lateral reticular nucleus
MF	mossy fiber
MGB	medial geniculate body
OFC	output feature cluster
PC	Purkinje cell
PF	parallel fiber
PN	pontine nucleus
VPL	ventroposterolateral
VL	ventral lateral
VOR	vestibuloocular reflex
VSR	vestibulospinal reflex

BIBLIOGRAPHY

This bibliography contains two types of entries: (1) citations given or work alluded to in the report, and (2) additional references to pertinent literature by conference participants and others. Citations in group (1) may be found in the text on the pages in the right-hand column.

Page

Adám, A. (1968): Simulation of rhythmic nervous activities. II. Mathematical models for the function of networks with cyclic inhibition. *Kybernetik* 5:103-109.

Adám, A. (1968): Uber stochastische Wahrheitsfunktionen. *In: Proceedings of the Colloquium on Information Theory, Vol. I.* Rényi, A., ed. Budapest: János Bolyai Mathematical Society, pp. 15-34.

Adám, A. (1971): On some generalizations of cyclic networks. *Acta Cybernetica* 1:106-119.

Adám, A. and Kling, U. (1971): On the behaviour of some cyclically symmetric networks. *Acta Cybernetica* 1:69-79.

Aizerman, M.A. and Andreeva, E.A. (1968a): Simple search mechanism for control   146
of skeletal muscles. *Automat. Remote Control* 29:452-463.

Aizerman, M.A. and Andreeva, E.A. (1968b): *On Some Control Mechanisms of*   146
Skeletal Muscles. Moscow: Institute of Automation and Remote Control.
(English and Russian versions.)

Aizerman, M.A. and Gurfinkel, V.S. (1970): *Issledovaniye protsessov upravleniya*   146
myshechnoy aktivnostyu (Investigations of Processes of Control of Muscular
Activity). Moscow: Nauka.

Andersen, P. and Eccles, J. (1962): Inhibitory phasing of neuronal discharge.   88,96
Nature 196:645-647.   119

Andersen, P., Eccles, J.C., and Sears, T.A. (1964): The ventro-basal complex of the   96
thalamus: types of cells, their responses and their functional organization.
J. Physiol. 174:370-399.

Andreeva, E.A., Turakhanov, K.A., Khutorskaya, O.E., and Chernov, V.I. (1969):   146
Connection between joint tremor and the joint angle control process. *Automat.*
Remote Control 30:1988-1993.

Anninos, P.A., Beek, B., Csermely, T.J., Harth, E.M., and Pertile, G. (1970):   51
Dynamics of neural structures. *J. Theor. Biol.* 26:121-148.

Arbib, M.A. (1969): *Theories of Abstract Automata.* Englewood Cliffs, N.J.:   26
Prentice-Hall, Inc.

Arbib, M.A. (1970): Cognition–a cybernetic approach. *In: Cognition: A Multiple View.* (Symposium on Cognitive Studies and Artificial Intelligence Research, University of Chicago, 1969.) Garvin, P.L., ed. New York: Spartan Books, pp. 331-348.

Arbib, M.A. (1971): How we know universals: retrospect and prospect. *Math. Biosci.* 11:95-107.

Arbib, M.A. (1972a): *The Metaphorical Brain: An Introduction to Cybernetics as*   8,9,26,
Artificial Intelligence and Brain Theory. New York: Wiley-Interscience.   38

Arbib, M.A. (1972b): Organization principles for theoretical neurophysiology. *In: Towards a Theoretical Biology, Vol. 4. Essays.* Waddington, C.H., ed. Edinburgh: Edinburgh University Press; Chicago: Aldine Publishing Co., pp. 146-168.

Arbib, M.A. (1972c): Toward an automata theory of brains. *Commun. Assoc. Comput. Mach.* 15:521-527.

Arbib, M.A., Boylls, C.C., and Dev, P. (1974): Neural models of spatial perception   121,159,
and the control of movement. *In: Cybernetics and Bionics.* Keidel, W.D.,   160,161,
Händler, W., and Spreng, M., eds. Munich: R. Oldenbourg, pp. 216-231.   163

Arbib, M.A. and Didday, R.L. (1971): The organization of action-oriented memory   24
for a perceiving system. Part 1: The basic model. *J. Cybernet.* 1:3-18.

Armstrong, D.M., Harvey, R.J., and Schild, R.F. (1973a): Cerebello-cerebellar   147
responses mediated via climbing fibres. *Exp. Brain Res.* 18:19-39.

Armstrong, D.M., Harvey, R.J., and Schild, R.F. (1973b): The spatial organisation   147
of climbing fibre branching in the cat cerebellum. *Exp. Brain Res.* 18:40-58.

Armstrong, D.M., Harvey, R.J., and Schild, R.F. (1973c): Spino-olivocerebellar   147
pathways to the posterior lobe of the cat cerebellum. *Exp. Brain Res.* 18:1-18.

Arshavskii, Y.I., Kots, Y.M., Orlovskii, G.N., Rodionov, I.N., and Shik, M.L.   165
(1965): Investigation of the biomechanics of running by the dog. *Biophysics* 10:737-746.

Arshavsky, Y.I., Berkinblit, M.B., Fukson, O.I., Gelfand, I.M., and Orlovsky, G.N.   148
(1972): Origin of modulation in neurones of the ventral spinocerebellar tract during locomotion. *Brain Res.* 43:276-279.

Asanuma, H. and Rosén, I. (1972): Topographical organization of cortical efferent   98
zones projecting to distal forelimb muscles in the monkey. *Exp. Brain Res.* 14:243-256.

Barlow, H.B., Blakemore, C., and Pettigrew, J.D. (1967): The neural mechanism of binocular depth discrimination. *J. Physiol.* 193:327-342.

Barlow, H.B. and Levick, W.R. (1965): The mechanism of directionally selective   85
units in rabbit's retina. *J. Physiol.* 178:477-504.

Bell, C.C. and Kawasaki, T. (1972): Relations among climbing fiber responses of   162
nearby Purkinje cells. *J. Neurophysiol.* 35:155-169.

Benevento, L.A., Creutzfeldt, O.D., and Kuhnt, U. (1972): Significance of   105,108
intracortical inhibition in the visual cortex. *Nature New Biol.* 238:124-126.

Bernstein, N. (1967): *The Co-ordination and Regulation of Movements.* Oxford: 157
Pergamon Press.

Beurle, R.L. (1954): Properties of a block of cells capable of regenerating pulses.   43,117
Royal Radar Establishment Memorandum 1043.

Beurle, R.L. (1956): Properties of a mass of cells capable of regenerating pulses.   117
Phil. Trans. Roy. Soc. B 240:55-94.

Blakemore, C. (1969): Binocular depth discrimination and the nasotemporal
division. *J. Physiol.* 205:471-497.

Blakemore, C. (1970a): Binocular depth perception and the optic chiasm. *Vision
Res.* 10:43-47.

Blakemore, C. (1970b): A new kind of stereoscopic vision. *Vision Res.*   22,112
10:1181-1199.

Blakemore, C. (1970c): The range and scope of binocular depth discrimination in
man. *J. Physiol.* 211:599-622.

Blakemore, C. (1970d): The representation of three-dimensional visual space in the
cat's striate cortex. *J. Physiol.* 209:155-178.

Blakemore, C. (1974): Developmental factors in the formation of feature extracting   114
neurons. *In: The Neurosciences: Third Study Program.* Schmitt, F.O. and
Worden, F.G., eds. Cambridge, Mass.: M.I.T. Press, pp. 105-113.

Blakemore, C., Carpenter, R.H.S., and Georgeson, M.A. (1970): Lateral inhibition   105,113
between orientation detectors in the human visual system. *Nature* 228:37-39.

Blakemore, C., Carpenter, R.H.S., and Georgeson, M.A. (1971): Lateral thinking
about lateral inhibition. *Nature* 234:418-419.

Blakemore, C. and Cooper, G.F. (1970): Development of the brain depends on the   114
visual environment. *Nature* 228:477-478.

Blakemore, C., Fiorentini, A., and Maffei, L. (1972): A second neural mechanism   112
of binocular depth discrimination. *J. Physiol.* 226:725-749.

Blakemore, C. and Hague, B. (1972): Evidence for disparity detecting neurones in
the human visual system. *J. Physiol.* 225:437-455.

Blakemore, C. and Julesz, B. (1971): Stereoscopic depth aftereffect produced
without monocular cues. *Science* 171:286-288.

Blakemore, C. and Mitchell, D.E. (1973): Environmental modification of the visual   114
cortex and the neural basis of learning and memory. *Nature* 241:467-468.

Blakemore, C. and Pettigrew, J.D. (1970): Eye dominance in the visual cortex.
Nature 225:426-429.

Blakemore, C. and Tobin, E.A. (1972): Lateral inhibition between orientation   105,108,
detectors in the cat's visual cortex. *Exp. Brain Res.* 15:439-440.   112

Blakemore, C. and Van Sluyters, R.C. (1974): Reversal of the physiological effects
of monocular deprivation in kittens: further evidence for a sensitive period.
J. Physiol. 237:195-216.

Bloedel, J.R. and Roberts, W.J. (1971): Action of climbing fibers in cerebellar
cortex of the cat. *J. Neurophysiol.* 34:17-31.

Bobrow, L. and Arbib, M.A. (1974): *Discrete Mathematics: Applied Algebra for*   40
Computer and Information Science. Philadelphia: W.B. Saunders Co.,
pp. 367-387.

Bodian, D. (1952): Introductory survey of neurons. *Cold Spring Harbor Symp.*   49
Quant. Biol. 17:1-13.

Bonin, G. von and Mehler, W.R. (1971): On columnar arrangement of nerve cells in
cerebral cortex. *Brain Res.* 27:1-9.

Boylls, C.C. (1975): A theory of cerebellar function with applications to   139,158
locomotion. COINS Technical Report. Amherst, Mass.: Computer and Information Science, University of Massachusetts. (In press)

Boylls, C.C. and Arbib, M.A. (1975): The cerebellum: a case study in brain theory.
Prog. Biophys. Mol. Biol. (In press)

Braitenberg, V. (1961): Functional interpretation of cerebellar histology. *Nature*   130
190:539-540.

Braitenberg, V. (1965a): Taxis, kinesis and decussation. *Prog. Brain Res.*   16
17:210-222.

Braitenberg, V. (1965b): What can be learned from spike interval histograms about
synaptic mechanisms. *J. Theor. Biol.* 8:419-425.

Braitenberg, V. (1967a): Is the cerebellar cortex a biological clock in the   130
millisecond range? *Prog. Brain Res.* 25:334-346.

Braitenberg, V. (1967b): Patterns of projection in the visual system of the fly.
I. Retina-lamina projections. *Exp. Brain Res.* 3:271-298.

Braitenberg, V. (1970): Ordnung und Orientierung der Elemente im Sehsystem der
Fliege. *Kybernetik* 7:235-242.

Braitenberg, V. (1973): *Gehirngespinste—Neuroanatomie für kybernetische Inter-*   130
essierte. New York: Springer-Verlag.

Braitenberg, V. (1974): Period structures and structural gradients in the visual ganglia of the fly. *In: Symposium Datenverarbeitung im visuellen System der Arthropoden, Zurich.* (In press)

Braitenberg, V. and Atwood, R.P. (1958): Morphological observations on the cerebellar cortex. *J. Comp. Neurol.* 109:1-33.   130

Braitenberg, V. and Kemali, M. (1970): Exceptions to bilateral symmetry in the epithalamus of lower vertebrates. *J. Comp. Neurol.* 138:137-146.

Braitenberg, V. and Onesto, N. (1960): The cerebellar cortex as a timing organ.   130
Discussion of an hypothesis. *In: Proceedings of the 1st International Conference on Medical Cybernetics.* Naples: Giannini, pp. 239-255.

Brodal, A., Lacerda, A.M., Destombes, J., and Angaut, P. (1972): The pattern in   160
the projection of the intracerebellar nuclei onto the nucleus reticularis tegmenti pontis in the cat. An experimental anatomical study. *Exp. Brain Res.* 16:140-160.

Brodal, A. and Szikla, G. (1972): The termination of the brachium conjunctivum   160
descendens in the nucleus reticularis tegmenti pontis. An experimental anatomical study in the cat. *Brain Res.* 39:337-351.

Brooks, V.B., Rudomin, P., and Slayman, C.L. (1961): Peripheral receptive fields of neurons in the cat's cerebral cortex. *J. Neurophysiol.* 24:302-325.

Brooks, V.B. and Wilson, V.J. (1959): Recurrent inhibition in the cat's spinal cord   96
J. Physiol. 146:380-391.

Brown, J.E. and Major, D. (1966): Cat retinal ganglion cell dendritic fields. *Exp.*   104
Neurol. 15:70-78.

Bullock, T.H. (1974): Comparisons between vertebrates and invertebrates in   39
nervous organization. *In: The Neurosciences: Third Study Program.* Schmitt, F.O. and Worden, F.G., eds. Cambridge, Mass.: M.I.T. Press, pp. 343-346.

Bullock, T.H. and Horridge, G.A. (1965): *Structure and Function in the Nervous*   43
Systems of Invertebrates, Vols. I and II. San Francisco: W.H. Freeman.

Bunge, R.P. and Bunge, M.B. (1965): Ultrastructural characteristics of synapses   50
forming in cultured spinal cord. *Anat. Rec.* 151:329. (Abstr.)

Burke, W. and Sefton, A.J. (1966): Inhibitory mechanisms in lateral geniculate nucleus of rat. *J. Physiol.* 187:231-246.

Burns, B.D. (1968): *The Uncertain Nervous System.* London: Edward Arnold Ltd.   112,120

Burns, B.D. and Pritchard, R. (1971): Geometrical illusions and the response of neurones in the cat's visual cortex to angle patterns. *J. Physiol.* 213:599-616.

Carraher, R.G. and Thurston, J.B. (1966): *Optical Illusions and the Visual Arts.*   99
New York: Van Nostrand Reinhold Co.

Chernov, V.I. (1968): Control over single muscles or a pair of muscle-antagonists   146
under conditions of precision search. *Automat. Remote Control* 29:1090-1101.

Chow, K.L. and Leiman, A.L. (1970): The structural and functional organization of   74
the neocortex. *Neurosciences Res. Prog. Bull.* 8:153-220. Also *In: Neurosciences Research Symposium Summaries, Vol. 5.* Schmitt, F.O. et al., eds.
Cambridge, Mass.: M.I.T. Press, 1971, pp. 149-213.

Cleland, B.G., Dubin, M.W., and Levick, W.R. (1971): Simultaneous recording of   104
input and output of lateral geniculate neurons. *Nature New Biol.* 231:191-192.

Colonnier, M.L. (1966): The structural design of the neocortex. *In: Brain and*   43,70,
Conscious Experience. Eccles, J.C., ed. New York: Springer-Verlag, pp. 1-23.   73

Colonnier, M. (1968): Synaptic patterns on different cell types in the different   70
laminae of the cat visual cortex. An electron microscope study. *Brain Res.*
9:268-287.

Colonnier, M. and Guillery, R.W. (1964): Synaptic organization in the lateral   86
geniculate nucleus of the monkey. *Z. Zellforsch. Mikrosk. Anat.* 62:333-355.

Cooke, J.D., Larson, B., Oscarsson, O., and Sjölund, B. (1971): Origin and   147
termination of cuneocerebellar tract. *Exp. Brain Res.* 13:339-358.

Cosgriff, R.L. (1958): *Nonlinear Control Systems.* New York: McGraw-Hill.   146

Cragg, B.G. and Temperley, H.N.V. (1954): The organisation of neurones: a   99
co-operative analogy. *Electroencephalogr. Clin. Neurophysiol.* 6:85-92.

Craik, K.J.W. (1943): *The Nature of Explanation.* Cambridge: Cambridge Univer-   8
sity Press.

Craik, K.J.W. (1966): The mechanism of human action. *In: The Nature of*   8
Psychology: A Selection of Papers, Essays and Other Writings by the late
Kenneth J.W. Craik. Sherwood, S.L., ed. Cambridge: Cambridge University
Press, pp. 7-90.

Crain, S.M. (1973a): Microelectrode recording in brain tissue cultures. *In: Methods*   50
in Physiological Psychology, Vol. I. Bioelectric Recording Techniques, Part A.
Thompson, R.F. and Patterson, M.M., eds. New York: Academic Press,
pp. 39-75.

Crain, S.M. (1973b): Tissue culture models of developing brain functions. *In:*   50
Developmental Studies of Behavior and the Nervous System. Vol. 2. Aspects of
Neurogenesis. New York: Academic Press, pp. 69-114.

Creutzfeldt, O.D. (1968): Physiologie der Hirnrinde. *Jahrb. Max-Planck Gesell-*   104
schaft: 61-89.

Creutzfeldt, O.D. (1970): Some principles of synaptic organization in the visual   57
system. *In: The Neurosciences: Second Study Program.* Schmitt, F.O.,
editor-in-chief. New York: Rockefeller University Press, pp. 630-647.

Creutzfeldt, O.D. (1972): Transfer function of the retina. *Electroencephalogr. Clin. Neurophysiol. Suppl.* 31:159-169.

Creutzfeldt, O., Noda, H., and Freeman, R.B., Jr. (1972): Neurophysiological   29
correlates of eye movements in the visual cortex. *Bibl. Opthalmol.* 82:199-206.

Creutzfeldt, O., Pöppl, E., and Singer, W. (1971): Quantitativer Ansatz zur Analyse   14,111
der funktionellen Organisation des visuellen Cortex (Untersuchungen an
Primaten). *In: Pattern Recognition in Biological and Technical Systems.*
(Proceedings of the 4th Congress of the Deutsche Gesellschaft für Kybernetik,
Berlin, Technical University, April 6-9, 1970.) Grüsser, O.-J. and Klinke, R., eds.
Heidelberg: Springer-Verlag, pp. 81-96.

Creutzfeldt, O. and Sakmann, B. (1969): Neurophysiology of vision. *Annu. Rev. Physiol.* 31:499-544.

Creutzfeldt, O.D., Sakmann, B., Scheich, H., and Korn, A. (1970): Sensitivity
distribution and spatial summation within receptive-field center of retinal
on-center ganglion cells and transfer function of the retina. *J. Neurophysiol.*
33:654-671.

Czéh, G. and Székely, G. (1971): Muscle activities recorded simultaneously from   63
normal and supernumerary forelimbs in ambystoma. *Acta Physiol. Acad. Sci.
Hung.* 40:287-301.

Dertouzos, M.L. (1967): PHASEPLOT: an on-line graphical display technique.   33
IEEE Trans. Electron. Comput. EC-16:203-209.

Dertouzos, M.L. and Graham, H.L. (1966): A parametric graphical display   33
technique for on-line use. *In: AFIPS Conference Proceedings, Vol. 29.* (Proceedings of the Fall Joint Computer Conference, Nov. 7-10, 1966, San
Francisco, Calif.) Washington, D.C.: Spartan Books, pp. 201-209.

Dev, P. (1974): Segmentation processes in visual perception: a cooperative neural   117,120
model. COINS Technical Report 74C-5. Amherst, Mass.: Computer and
Information Science, University of Massachusetts.

Didday, R.L. (1970): The simulation and modeling of distributed information   26,27
processing in the frog visual system. Ph.D. Thesis, Information Systems
Laboratory, Stanford University, Stanford, Calif.

Didday, R.L. and Arbib, M.A. (1973): Eye movements and visual perception: a   23,24,26
"two visual system" model. COINS Technical Report 73C-9. Amherst, Mass.:
Computer and Information Science, University of Massachusetts.

Dressler, R.M. (1967): An approach to model-referenced adaptive control systems.   36
IEEE Trans. Automatic Control AC-12:75-80.

Dreyer, D.A., Schneider, R.J., Metz, C.B., and Whitsel, B.L. (1974): Differential   19
contributions of spinal pathways to body representation in postcentral gyrus of
Macaca mulatta. J. Neurophysiol. 37:119-145.

Dubner, R. and Zeki, S.M. (1971): Response properties and receptive fields of cells   21
in an anatomically defined region of the superior temporal sulcus in the
monkey. *Brain Res.* 35:528-532.

Duffy, F.H. and Burchfiel, J.L. (1971): Somatosensory systems: Organizational   20,21
hierarchy from single units in monkey area 5. *Science* 172:273-275.

Eccles, J. (1965): Functional meaning of the patterns of synaptic connections in   44
the cerebellum. *Perspect. Biol. Med.* 8:289-310.

Eccles, J.C. (1967): Circuits in the cerebellar control of movement. *Proc. Nat.*   144
Acad. Sci. 58:336-343.

Eccles, J.C. (1969a): The development of the cerebellum of vertebrates in relation
to the control of movement. *Naturwissenschaften* 56:525-534.

Eccles, J.C. (1969b): The dynamic loop hypothesis of movement control. *In:*   146
Information Processing in the Nervous System. (Proceedings of a Symposium
held at the State University of New York at Buffalo, Oct. 21-24, 1968.)
Liebovic, K.N., ed. New York: Springer-Verlag, pp. 245-269.

Eccles, J.C. (1971): Functional significance of arrangement of neurones in cell   154
assemblies. *Arch. Psychiatr. Nervenkr.* 215:92-106.

Eccles, J.C. (1973a): The cerebellum as a computer: patterns in space and time.   145
J. Physiol. 229:1-32.

Eccles, J.C. (1973b): *The Understanding of the Brain.* New York: McGraw-Hill.   127,128,
                                                                                         141,142
Eccles, J.C., Faber, D.S., Murphy, J.T., Sabah, N.H., and Táboříková, H. (1969):
Firing patterns of Purkinje cells in response to volleys from limb nerves. *Brain*
Res. 14:222-226.

Eccles, J.C., Faber, D.S., Murphy, J.T., Sabah, N.H., and Táboříková, H. (1971a):
Afferent volleys in limb nerves influencing impulse discharges in cerebellar
cortex. I. In mossy fibers and granule cells. *Exp. Brain Res.* 13:15-35.

Eccles, J.C., Faber, D.S., Murphy, J.T., Sabah, N.H., and Táboříková, H. (1971b):
Afferent volleys in limb nerves influencing impulse discharges in cerebellar
cortex. II. In Purkyně cells. *Exp. Brain Res.* 13:36-53.

Eccles, J.C., Faber, D.S., Murphy, J.T., Sabah, N.H., and Táboříková, H. (1971c):   70,128
Investigations on integration of mossy fiber inputs to Purkyně cells in the
anterior lobe. *Exp. Brain Res.* 13:54-77.

Eccles, J.C., Fatt, P., and Koketsu, K. (1954a): Cholinergic and inhibitory synapses   44,96
in a pathway from motor-axon collaterals to motoneurones. *J. Physiol.*
126:524-562.

Eccles, J.C., Fatt, P., and Landgren, S. (1956): Central pathway for direct
inhibitory action of impulses in largest afferent nerve fibres to muscle.
J. Neurophysiol. 19:75-98.

Eccles, J.C., Fatt, P., Landgren, S., and Winsbury, G.J. (1954b): Spinal cord 44
potentials generated by volleys in the large muscle afferents. *J. Physiol.*
125:590-606.

Eccles, J.C., Ito, M., and Szentágothai, J. (1967): *The Cerebellum as a Neuronal* 44,54,65,
Machine. New York: Springer-Verlag. 66,69,131,
143,154,156
Eccles, J.C., Provini, L., Strata, P., and Táboříková, H. (1968a): Analysis of
electrical potentials evoked in the cerebellar anterior lobe by stimulation of
hindlimb and forelimb nerves. *Exp. Brain Res.* 6:171-194.

Eccles, J.C., Provini, L., Strata, P., and Táboříková, H. (1968b): Topographical
investigations on the climbing fiber inputs from forelimb and hindlimb afferents
to the cerebellar anterior lobe. *Exp. Brain Res.* 6:195-215.

Eccles, J.C., Rosén, I., Scheid, P., and Táboříková, H. (1972a): Cutaneous afferent
responses in interpositus neurones of the cat. *Brain Res.* 42:207-211.

Eccles, J.C., Sabah, N.H., Schmidt, R.F., and Táboříková, H. (1971d): Cerebellar
Purkyně cell responses to cutaneous mechanoreceptors. *Brain Res.* 30:419-424.

Eccles, J.C., Sabah, N.H., Schmidt, R.F., and Táboříková, H. (1972b): Cutaneous
mechanoreceptors influencing impulse discharges in cerebellar cortex. I. In
mossy fibers. *Exp. Brain Res.* 15:245-260.

Eccles, J.C., Sabah, N.H., Schmidt, R.F., and Táboříková, H. (1972c): Cutaneous
mechanoreceptors influencing impulse discharges in cerebellar cortex. II. In
Purkyně cells by mossy fiber input. *Exp. Brain Res.* 15:261-277.

Eccles, J.C., Sabah, N.H., Schmidt, R.F., and Táboříková, H. (1972d): Cutaneous 149
mechanorecpetors influencing impulse discharges in cerebellar cortex. III. In
Purkyně cells by climbing fiber input. *Exp. Brain Res.* 15:484-497.

Eccles, J.C., Sabah, N.H., Schmidt, R.F., and Táboříková, H. (1972e): Integration 149,151
by Purkyně cells of mossy and climbing fiber inputs from cutaneous
mechanoreceptors. *Exp. Brain Res.* 15:498-520.

Eccles, J.C., Sabah, N.H., Schmidt, R.F., and Táboříková, H. (1972f): Mode of
operation of the cerebellum in the dynamic loop control of movement. *Brain
Res.* 40:73-80.

Eccles, J.C., Sabah, N.H., and Táboříková, H. (1971e): Responses evoked in
neurones of the fastigial nucleus by cutaneous mechanoreceptors. *Brain Res.*
35:523-527.

Economo, C.F. von and Koskinas, G.N. (1925): *Die Cytoarchitektonik der* 44
Hirnrinde des erwachsenen Menschen. Vienna: Springer-Verlag.

Edds, M.V., Jr., Barkley, D.S., and Fambrough, D.M. (1972): Genesis of neuronal
patterns. *Neurosciences Res. Prog. Bull.* 10:262-268. Also *In: Neurosciences
Research Symposium Summaries, Vol. 7.* Schmitt, F.O. et al., eds. Cambridge,
Mass.: M.I.T. Press, 1973, pp. 262-268.

Eidelberg, E. and Stein, D.G. (1974): Functional recovery after lesions of the
nervous system. *Neurosciences Res. Prog. Bull.* 12:191-303.

Ekerot, C.F. and Larson, B. (1972): Differential termination of the exteroceptive   150
and proprioceptive components of the cuneocerebellar tract. *Brain Res.*
36:420-424.

Ekerot, C.-F. and Larson, B. (1973): Correlation between sagittal projection zones   149,150,
of climbing and mossy fibre paths in cat cerebellar anterior lobe. *Brain Res.*   151
64:446-450.

Elias, H., Hennig, A., and Schwartz, D.E. (1971): Stereology: Applications to
biomedical research. *Physiol. Rev.* 51:158-200.

Elias, H. and Schwartz, D. (1971): Cerebro-cortical surface areas, volumes, lengths
of gyri and their interdependence in mammals, including man. *Z. Saeugetierk.*
36:147-163.

Erulkar, S.D., Butler, R.A., and Gerstein, G.L. (1968): Excitation and inhibition in   56,85
cochlear nucleus. II. Frequency-modulated tones. *J. Neurophysiol.* 31:537-548.

Evans, E.F. (1968): Cortical representation. *In: Hearing Mechanisms in Vertebrates.*   21,22
(A Ciba Foundation Symposium.) De Reuck, A.V.S. and Knight, J., eds.
Boston, Mass.: Little, Brown and Co., pp. 272-295.

Evarts, E.V. (1967): Representation of movements and muscles by pyramidal tract
neurons of the precentral motor cortex. *In: Neurophysiological Basis of Normal
and Abnormal Motor Activities.* (Proceedings of the Third Symposium of the
Parkinson's Disease Information and Research Center of Columbia University,
Nov. 28-29, 1966.) Yahr, M.D. and Purpura, D.P., eds. Hewlett, N.Y.: Raven
Press, pp. 215-253.

Evarts, E.V. (1968): Relation of pyramidal tract activity to force exerted during
voluntary movement. *J. Neurophysiol.* 31:14-27.

Evarts, E.V., Bizzi, E., Burke, R.E., DeLong, M., and Thach, W.T., Jr. (1971):   11,27,29,
Central control of movement. *Neurosciences Res. Prog. Bull.* 9:1-170. Also *In:* 37,38,91,
Neurosciences Research Symposium Summaries, Vol. 6. Schmitt, F.O. et al.,   98,148
eds. Cambridge, Mass.: M.I.T. Press, 1972, pp. 1-170.

Famiglietti, E.V., Jr. and Peters, A. (1972): The synaptic glomerulus and the   86,88
intrinsic neuron in the dorsal lateral geniculate nucleus of the cat. *J. Comp.
Neurol.* 144:285-333.

Farley, B.G. (1964): The use of computer technics in neural research. *In: Neural*   43
Theory and Modeling. (Proceedings of the 1962 Ojai Symposium.) Reiss, R.F.,
ed. Stanford, Calif.: Stanford University Press, pp. 43-72.

Fender, D. and Julesz, B. (1967): Extension of Panum's fusional area in binocularly 103,120
stabilized vision. *J. Opt. Soc. Am.* 57:819-830.

Ferrando, F.R. (1962): Information, entropy, and nervous system. *Perspect. Biol.
Med.* 5:296-307.

Bibliography

Forssberg, H. and Grillner, S. (1973): The locomotion of the acute spinal cat injected with clonidine i.v. *Brain Res.* 50:184-186. 158

Fox, C.A. (1962): The structure of the cerebellar cortex. *In: Correlative Anatomy of the Nervous System.* Crosby, E.C., Humphrey, T., and Lauer, E.W., eds. New York: Crowell-Collier and Macmillan, pp. 193-198. 126

Freeman, J.A. (1969): The cerebellum as a timing device: an experimental study in the frog. *In: Neurobiology of Cerebellar Evolution and Development.* Llinás, R., ed. Chicago: American Medical Assoc., pp. 397-420. 130

Fuster, J.M., Creutzfeldt, O.D., and Straschill, M. (1965): Intracellular recording of neuronal activity in the visual system. *Z. Vergl. Physiol.* 49:605-622. 104

Gazzaniga, M.S. (1970): *The Bisected Brain.* New York: Appleton-Century-Crofts, Inc. 16

Gelfand, I.M., Gurfinkel, V.S., Tsetlin, M.L., and Shik, M.L. (1971): Some problems in the analysis of movements. *In: Models of the Structural-Functional Organization of Certain Biological Systems.* Gelfand, I.M., Gurfinkel, V.S., Fomin, S.V., and Tsetlin, M.L., eds. Cambridge, Mass.: M.I.T. Press, pp. 329-345. 35,157

Gerlach, J. (1872): Ueber die Struktur der grauen Substanz des menschlichen Grosshirns. Vorläufige Mittheilung. *Zentralbl. Med. Wiss.* 10:273-275. 42

Gibson, J.J. (1962): Observations on active touch. *Psychol. Rev.* 69:477-491. 18

Globus, A. and Scheibel, A.B. (1967): Pattern and field in cortical structure: the rabbit. *J. Comp. Neurol.* 131:155-172. 58,74,79

Gonshor, A. and Melvill Jones, G. (1973): Changes of human vestibulo-ocular response induced by vision-reversal during head rotation. *J. Physiol.* 234:102P-103P. 135,140

Götz, K.G. (1968): Flight control in *Drosophila* by visual perception of motion. *Kybernetik* 4:199-208. 29

Graham, D. and McRuer, D.T. (1961): *Analysis of Nonlinear Control Systems.* New York: John Wiley and Sons, Inc., pp. 323-324, 345-354. 146

Granit, R. and Phillips, C.G. (1956): Excitatory and inhibitory processes acting upon individual Purkinje cells of the cerebellum in cats. *J. Physiol.* 133:520-547. 126

Greene, P.H. (1969): Seeking mathematical models for skilled actions. *In: Biomechanics.* (Proceedings of the First Rock Island Arsenal Biomechanics Symposium, April 5-6, 1967.) Bootzin, D. and Muffley, H.C., eds. New York: Plenum Press, pp. 149-180. 33,62

Greene, P.H. (1971): Introduction. *In: Models of the Structural-Functional Organization of Certain Biological Systems.* Gelfand, I.M., Gurfinkel, V.S., Fomin, S.V., and Tsetlin, M.L., eds. Cambridge, Mass.: M.I.T. Press, pp. xi-xxxi. 33

Page

Greene, P.H. (1972): Problems of organization of motor systems. *In: Progress in*   33,34,
Theoretical Biology, Vol. 2. Rosen, R. and Snell, F.M., eds. New York: 146
Academic Press, pp. 303-338.

Greene, P.H. (1973a): Cooperation of effectors. Institute for Task Analysis   33
Memorandum No. 14. Chicago: Center for Control Research, 1357 E. 57 Street.

Greene, P.H. (1973b): Coordination of effectors. Institute for Task Analysis   33
Memorandum No. 15. Chicago: Center for Control Research, 1357 E. 57 Street.

Greene, P.H. (1973c): Hierarchical hybrid control of manipulators, artificial
intelligence in LSI. *In: Remotely Manned Systems. Exploration and Operation*
in Space. (Proceedings of 1st National Conference, California Institute of
Technology, Pasadena, Calif., Sept. 13-15, 1972.) Heer, E., ed. Pasadena, Calif.:
California Institute of Technology Press, pp. 431-446.

Greene, P.H. (1973d): Organization of hierarchical control systems. Institute for   33
Task Analysis Memorandum No. 17. Chicago: Center for Control Research,
1357 E. 57 Street.

Greene, P.H. (1975a): Proposed organization of hierarchical multicomputer control   33
system. *Int. J. Man-Machine Stud.* (In press)

Greene, P.H. (1975b): User's guide to generation 4½ multicomputer systems. *Int.*   33
J. Man-Machine Stud. (In press)

Gregory, R.L. (1969): On how so little information controls so much behaviour.   8
In: Towards a Theoretical Biology. Vol. 2. Sketches. (An International Union of
Biological Sciences Symposium.) Waddington, C.H., ed. Edinburgh: Edinburgh
University Press; Chicago: Aldine Publishing Co., pp. 236-247.

Grillner, S. and Shik, M.L. (1973): On the descending control of the lumbosacral   158
spinal cord from the "mesencephalic locomotor region." *Acta Physiol. Scand.*
87:320-333.

Grüsser, O.-J. (1972): Informationstheorie und die Signalverarbeitung in den
Sinnesorganen und im Nervensystem. *Naturwissenschaften* 59:436-447.

Guillery, R.W. (1966): A study of Golgi preparations from the dorsal lateral   58
geniculate nucleus of the adult cat. *J. Comp. Neurol.* 128:21-49.

Guillery, R.W. (1969): The organization of synaptic interconnections in the
laminae of the dorsal lateral geniculate nucleus of the cat. *Z. Zellforsch.*
Mikrosk. Anat. 96:1-38.

Hajdu, F., Somogyi, G., and Tombol, T. (1974): Neuronal and synaptic   87
arrangement in the lateralis posterior-pulvinar complex of the thalamus in the
cat. *Brain Res.* 73:89-104.

Hámori, J. (1973): Developmental morphology of dendritic postsynaptic specializa-   68
tions. *In: Recent Developments of Neurobiology in Hungary, Vol. IV. Results in*
Neuroanatomy, Neuroendocrinology, Neurophysiology and Behaviour, Neuro-
pathology. Lissák, K., ed. Budapest: Akadémiai Kiadó, pp. 9-32.

Bibliography

Hámori, J., Pasik, P., Pasik, T., and Szentágothai, J. (1975): "Triadic" synaptic   89
arrangements and their possible significance in the lateral geniculate nucleus of
the monkey. *Brain Res.* (In press)

Hámori, J. and Szentágothai, J. (1964): The "crossing over" synapse: An electron   52
microscope study of the molecular layer in the cerebellar cortex. *Acta Biol.
Acad. Sci. Hung.* 15:95-117.

Harrison, J.M. and Irving, R. (1966): The organization of the posterior ventral   56,57
cochlear nucleus in the rat. *J. Comp. Neurol.* 126:391-401.

Harth, E.M., Csermely, T.J., Beek, B., and Lindsay, R.D. (1970): Brain functions   51
and neural dynamics. *J. Theor. Biol.* 26:93-120.

Hartline, H.K. and Ratliff, F. (1957): Inhibitory interaction of receptor units in the
eye of *Limulus. J. Gen. Physiol.* 40:357-376.

Hebb, D. (1949): *The Organization of Behavior.* New York: John Wiley and Sons,   113
Inc.

Helmholtz, H. (1867): *Handbuch der Physiologischen Optik.* Leipzig: Leopold   127
Voss. (English translation in 1925: *Treatise on Physiological Optics, Vol. III.
The Perceptions of Vision.* Southall, J.P.C., ed. Washington, D.C.: The Optical
Society of America.)

Henneman, E. (1971): Over what range of normal movement may we expect
Henneman's "size principle" to operate? *Neurosciences Res. Prog. Bull.*
9:127-129. Also *In: Neurosciences Research Symposium Summaries, Vol. 6.*
Schmitt, F.O. et al., eds. Cambridge, Mass.: M.I.T. Press, 1972, pp. 127-129.

Henry, G.H. and Bishop, P.O. (1971): Simple cells of the striate cortex. *In:
Contributions to Sensory Physiology, Vol. 5.* Neff, W.D., ed. New York:
Academic Press, pp. 1-46.

Herndon, R.M., Margolis, G., and Kilham, L. (1969): Virus induced cerebellar
malformation. An electron microscopic study. *J. Neuropathol. Exp. Neurol.*
28:164. (Abstr.)

Hirsch, H.V.B. and Spinelli, D.N. (1971): Modification of the distribution of   113
receptive field orientation in cats by selective visual exposure during development. *Exp. Brain Res.* 12:509-527.

Holmes, G. (1939): The cerebellum of man. *Brain* 62:1-30.   125

Hubel, D.H. and Wiesel, T.N. (1962): Receptive fields, binocular interaction and   45,109,
functional architecture in the cat's visual cortex. *J. Physiol.* 160:106-154.   111

Hubel, D.H. and Wiesel, T.N. (1963): Shape and arrangement of columns in cat's   45,105,
striate cortex. *J. Physiol.* 165:559-568.   106

Hubel, D.H. and Wiesel, T.N. (1965): Receptive fields and functional architecture   45,111
in two nonstriate visual areas (18 and 19) of the cat. *J. Neurophysiol.*
28:229-289.

Hubel, D.H. and Wiesel, T.N. (1968): Receptive fields and functional architecture   22,111
of monkey striate cortex. *J. Physiol.* 195:215-243.

Hubel, D.H. and Wiesel, T.N. (1970): Stereoscopic vision in macaque monkey. Cells   21,112
sensitive to binocular depth in area 18 of the macaque monkey cortex. *Nature*
225:41-42.

Hultborn, H., Jankowska, E., and Lindström, S. (1971): Relative contribution from   96,97
different nerves to recurrent depression of Ia IPSPs in motoneurones. *J. Physiol.*
215:637-664.

Ingle, D. and Sprague, J.M. (1975): Sensorimotor function of the midbrain tectum.   80
Neurosciences Res. Prog. Bull. 13:167-288.

Ito, M. (1970): Neurophysiological aspects of the cerebellar motor control system.   133
Int. J. Neurol. 7:162-176.

Ito, M. (1972a): Cerebellar control of the vestibular neurones: Physiology and   36,133
pharmacology. *Prog. Brain Res.* 37:377-390.

Ito, M. (1972b): Neural design of the cerebellar motor control system. *Brain Res.*   36,133
40:81-84.

Ito, M. (1973): The vestibulo-cerebellar relationships: Vestibulo-ocular reflex arc   137,138
and flocculus. *In: Handbook of Sensory Physiology, Vol. 6. Vestibular System.*
(Proceedings of a Symposium on the Vestibular System, April, 1973, University
of Chicago.) Kornhuber, H.H., ed. New York: Springer-Verlag, p. 25.

Ito, M. (1974): The control mechanisms of cerebellar motor systems. *In: The*   36,133,
Neurosciences: Third Study Program. Schmitt, F.O. and Worden, F.G., eds.   134,135,
Cambridge, Mass.: M.I.T. Press, pp. 293-303.   136,140

Jansen, J. and Brodal, A. (1940): Experimental studies on the intrinsic fibers of the   153
cerebellum. II. The cortico-nuclear projection. *J. Comp. Neurol.* 73:267-321.

Jansen, J. and Brodal, A. (1942): Experimental studies on the intrinsic fibers of the   153
cerebellum. The cortico-nuclear projection in the rabbit and the monkey
(*Macacus rhesus*). *Avh. Norske Vid.-Akad. I. Mat.-Nat. Kl.* No. 3:1-50.

Jones, E.G. and Powell, T.P.S. (1969): Electron microscopy of synaptic glomeruli
in the thalamic relay nuclei of the cat. *Proc. Roy. Soc. B* 172:153-171.

Jones, E.G. and Powell, T.P.S. (1970): An anatomical study of converging sensory   20
pathways within the cerebral cortex of the monkey. *Brain* 93:793-820.

Julesz, B. (1968): Experiment in perception. *Psychol. Today* 2(2):16-23.   102

Julesz, B. (1971): A holistic model. *In: Foundations of Cyclopean Perception.*   101,102,
Chicago: University of Chicago Press, pp. 186-220.   115,116,133

Jung, R. (1961): Neuronal integration in the visual cortex and its significance for   109
visual information. *In: Sensory Communication.* Rosenblith, W.A., ed.
Cambridge, Mass.: M.I.T. Press: New York: John Wiley and Sons, Inc.,
pp. 627-674.

Bibliography

Katchalsky, A. Katzir, Rowland, V., and Blumenthal, R. (1974): Dynamic patterns   119
of brain cell assemblies. *Neurosciences Res. Prog. Bull.* 12:1-187.

Kauffman, S. (1970a): Behaviour of randomly constructed genetic nets: binary   51
element nets. *In: Towards a Theoretical Biology, Vol. 3. Drafts.* (An International Union of Biological Sciences Symposium.) Waddington, C.H., ed.
Edinburgh: Edinburgh University Press, Chicago: Aldine Publishing Co.,
pp. 18-37.

Kauffman, S. (1970b): Behaviour of randomly constructed genetic nets: continuous
element nets. *In: Towards a Theoretical Biology, Vol. 3. Drafts.* (An International Union of Biological Sciences Symposium.) Waddington, C.H., ed.
Edinburgh: Edinburgh University Press; Chicago: Aldine Publishing Co.,
pp. 38-44.

Kelly, J.P. and Van Essen, D.C. (1974): Cell structure and function in the visual
cortex of the cat. *J. Physiol.* 238:515-547.

Kilmer, W.L., McCulloch, W.S., and Blum, J. (1968): Some mechanisms for a
theory of the reticular formation. *In: Systems Theory and Biology.* (Proceedings
of the III Systems Symposium at Case Institute of Technology.) Mesarović,
M.D., ed. New York: Springer-Verlag, pp. 286-375.

Kilmer, W.L., McCulloch, W.S., and Blum, J. (1969): A model of the vertebrate   49
central command system. *Int. J. Man-Machine Stud.* 1:279-309.

Kling, U. and Székely, G. (1968): Simulation of rhythmic nervous activities.
I. Function of networks with cyclic inhibitions. *Kybernetik* 5:89-103.

Korn, A. and Scheich, H. (1971): Übertragungseigenschaften der Katzenretina.
Kybernetik 8:179-188.

Kornhuber, H.H. (1971): Motor functions of cerebellum and basal ganglia: the   130
cerebellocortical saccadic (ballistic) clock, the cerebellonuclear hold regulator,
and the basal ganglia ramp (voluntary speed smooth movement) generator.
Kybernetik 8:157-162.

Kots, Y.N. and Syrovegin, A.V. (1966): Fixed set of variants of interaction of the   164
muscles of two joints used in the execution of simple voluntary movements.
Biophysics 11:1212-1219.

Land, M.F. (1974): A comparison of the visual behavior of a predatory arthropod   80
with that of a mammal. *In: The Neurosciences: Third Study Program.* Schmitt,
F.O. and Worden, F.G., eds. Cambridge, Mass.: M.I.T. Press, pp. 411-418.

Lázár, G. and Székely, G. (1967): Golgi studies on the optic center of the frog.   57
J. Hirnforsch. 9:329-344.

Legéndy, C.R. (1967): On the scheme by which the human brain stores   51
information. *Math. Biosci.* 1:555-597.

Leicht, R., Rowe, M.J., and Schmidt, R.F. (1973): Cutaneous convergence on to   149
the climbing fibre input to cerebellar Purkyně cells. *J. Physiol.* 228:601-618.

Page

Leontovich, T.A. and Zhukova, G.P. (1963): The specificity of the neuronal   49
structure and topography of the reticular formation in the brain and spinal cord
of carnivora. *J. Comp. Neurol.* 121:347-379.

Lettvin, J.Y., Maturana, H.R., McCulloch, W.S., and Pitts, W.H. (1959): What the   77
frog's eye tells the frog's brain. *Proc. IRE* 47:1940-1951.

Le Vay, S. (1971): On the neurons and synapses of the lateral geniculate nucleus of   88
the monkey, and the effects of eye enucleation. *Z. Zellforsch. Mikrosk. Anat.*
113:396-419.

Levick, W.R., Cleland, B.G., and Dubin, M.W. (1972): Lateral geniculate neurons of   104
cat: retinal inputs and physiology. *Invest. Ophthalmol.* 11:302-311.

Lindström, S. (1973): Recurrent control from motor axon collaterals of Ia   148
inhibitory pathways in the spinal cord of the cat. *Acta Physiol. Scand.*
392(Suppl.):3-93.

Llinás, R. (1970): Neuronal operations in cerebellar transactions. *In: The*   160
Neurosciences: Second Study Program. Schmitt, F.O., editor-in-chief. New
York: Rockefeller University Press, pp. 409-426.

Llinás, R. (1974): Motor aspects of cerebellar control. (Eighteenth Bowditch   93
Lecture.) *Physiologist* 17:19-46.

Llinás, R., Baker, R., and Sotelo, C. (1973): Electrical transmission between cells in   156
the inferior olive of the cat. *In: Program and Abstracts, Society for*
Neuroscience. Third Annual Meeting, San Diego, Calif., p. 156.

Llinás, R. and Hillman, D.E. (1969): Physiological and morphological organization   71
of the cerebellar circuits in various vertebrates. *In: Neurobiology of Cerebellar*
Evolution and Development. (Proceedings of the First International Symposium
of the Institute for Biomedical Research, American Medical Association/
Education and Research Foundation.) Llinás, R., ed. Chicago: American
Medical Assoc., pp. 43-73.

Llinás, R., Precht, W., and Clarke, M. (1971): Cerebellar Purkinje cell responses to   70,128
physiological stimulation of the vestibular system in the frog. *Exp. Brain Res.*
13:408-431.

Llinás, R. and Volkind, R.A. (1973): The olivo-cerebellar system: Functional
properties as revealed by harmaline-induced tremor. *Exp. Brain Res.* 18:69-87.

Loeb, J.M. (1952): A general linearizing process for non-linear control systems. *In:* 146
Automatic and Manual Control. (Papers contributed to the Conference at
Cranfield, 1951.) Tustin, A., ed. London: Butterworth, Inc., pp. 275-283.

Lorente de Nó, R. (1922): La corteza cerebral del ratón. (Primera contribución. La   43,108
corteza acústica.) *Trab. Lab. Invest. Biol. Univ. Madrid* 20:41-78.

Lorente de No, R. (1931): Ausgewahlte Kapitel aus der vergleichenden Physiologie   135
des Labyrinthes. Die Augenmuskelreflexe beim Kaninchen und ihre Grundlagen.
Ergeb. Physiol. 32:73-242.

Bibliography

183

Page

Lorente de Nó, R. (1932): The regulation of eye positions and movements induced by the labyrinth. *Laryngoscope* 42:233-330. — 43

Lorente de Nó, R. (1933): Vestibulo-ocular reflex arc. *Arch. Neurol. Psychiatr.* 30:245-291. — 43,44,79, 95

Lorente de Nó, R. (1938): Analysis of the activity of the chains of internuncial neurons. *J. Neurophysiol.* 1:207-244. — 43,44

Lundberg, A. (1969): *Reflex Control of Stepping.* (Norwegian Academy of Science and Letters, No. 5. The Nansen Memorial Lecture, Oct. 10, 1968.) Oslo: Universitetsforlaget.

Lundberg, A. (1970): The excitatory control of the Ia inhibitory pathway. *In: Excitatory Synaptic Mechanisms.* (Proceedings of the Fifth International Meeting of Neurobiologists, Sandefjord, Norway, Sept. 15-17, 1969.) Andersen, P. and Jansen, J.K.S., eds. Oslo: Universitetsforlaget, pp. 333-340. — 97

Lundberg, A. (1971): Function of the ventral spinocerebellar tract. A new hypothesis. *Exp. Brain Res.* 12:317-330. — 97,148

MacColl, L.A. (1945): Servomechanisms with alternating current motors and oscillating control servomechanisms. *In: Fundamental Theory of Servomechanisms.* New York: Van Nostrand Reinhold Co., pp. 73-87. — 146

McCulloch, W.S. (1945): A heterarchy of values determined by the topology of nervous nets. *Bull. Math. Biophys.* 7:89-93. — 14

McCulloch, W.S. (1965): *Embodiments of Mind.* Cambridge, Mass.: M.I.T. Press.

McCulloch, W.S. and Kilmer, W.L. (1969): Information processing in the central nervous system with special reference to the reticular system. *Ann. N.Y. Acad. Sci.* 161:416-419.

MacKay, D.M. (1956): The epistemological problem for automata. *In: Automata Studies.* Shannon, C.E. and McCarthy, J., eds. Princeton, N.J.: Princeton University Press, pp. 235-251. — 8

MacKay, D.M. (1957): Moving visual images produced by regular stationary patterns. *Nature* 180:849-850.

MacKay, D.M. (1962): Theoretical models of space perception. *In: Aspects of the Theory of Artificial Intelligence.* (Proceedings of the First International Symposium on Biosimulation, Locarno, June 29-July 5, 1960.) Muses, C.A., ed. New York: Plenum Press, pp. 83-103.

MacKay, D.M. (1963): Internal representation of the external world. *In: Proceedings of the AGARD Symposium on Natural and Artificial Logic Processors.* (Symposium held in Athens, Greece, 1963.) — 8

MacKay, D.M. (1965): Cerebral organization and the conscious control of action. *In: Brain and Conscious Experience.* (Study week, Sept. 28-Oct. 4, 1964, of the Pontificia Academia Scientiarum.) Eccles, J.C., ed. New York: Springer-Verlag, pp. 422-445. — 28

MacKay, D.M. and Mittelstaedt, H. (1974): Visual stability and motor control   29
(reafference revisited). *In: Cybernetics and Bionics.* Keidel, W.D., Händler, W.,
and Spreng, M., eds. Munich: R. Oldenbourg, pp. 71-80.

Maekawa, K. and Natsui, T. (1973): Climbing fiber activation of Purkinje cells in   137,140
rabbit's flocculus during light stimulation of the retina. *Brain Res.* 59:417-420.

Maekawa, K. and Simpson, J.I. (1972): Climbing fiber activation of Purkinje cells in   136
the flocculus by impulses transferred through the visual pathway. *Brain Res.*
39:245-251.

Maekawa, K. and Simpson, J.I. (1973): Climbing fiber responses evoked in   136
vestibulocerebellum of rabbit from visual system. *J. Neurophysiol.* 36:649-666.

Malsburg, C. von der (1973): Self-organization of orientation sensitive cells in the   113,124
striate cortex. *Kybernetik* 14:85-100.

Mannen, H. (1960): "Noyau fermé" et "noyau ouvert." Contribution à l'étude   155
cytoarchitectonique du tronc cérébral envisagée du point de vue du mode
d'arborisation dendritique. *Arch. Ital. Biol.* 98:333-350.

Mannen, H. (1969): A new approach for following the total course of the axon of   61
an individual neuron in Golgi-stained successive serial sections. Preliminary
report. *Proc. Jap. Acad.* 45:633-638.

Marin-Padilla, M. (1970): Prenatal and early postnatal ontogenesis of the human   70
motor cortex: A Golgi study. II. The basket-pyramidal system. *Brain Res.*
23:185-191.

Marr, D. (1969): A theory of cerebellar cortex. *J. Physiol.* 202:437-470.   117,131,135

Martinez, F.E., Crill, W.E., and Kennedy, T.T. (1970): Dendritic origin of climbing
fiber responses in cat cerebellar Purkinje cells. *Fed. Proc.* 29:324. (Abstr.)

Maturana, H.R., Lettvin, J.Y., McCulloch, W.S., and Pitts, W.H. (1960): Anatomy   57
and physiology of vision in the frog (*Rana pipiens*). *J. Gen. Physiol.* 43(Suppl.):
129-175.

Mendell, L.M. and Henneman, E. (1971): Terminals of single Ia fibers: Location,   53,59
density, and distribution within a pool of 300 homonymous motoneurons.
J. Neurophysiol. 34:171-187.

Merton, P.A., Morton, H.B., and Rashbass, C. (1967): Visual feedback in hand   146
tremor. *Nature* 216:583-584.

Metzler, J. and Spinelli, D.N. (1975): Behavioral correlates of physiological changes   114
produced in the activity of single units in the visual cortex of adult cats by
restricted, prolonged visual experience. *Brain Res.* (In press)

Milner, B. (1974): Hemispheric specialization: scope and limits. *In: The Neuro-*   16
sciences: Third Study Program. Schmitt, F.O. and Worden, F.G., eds.
Cambridge, Mass.: M.I.T. Press, pp. 75-89.

Minsky, M. (1961): Steps toward artificial intelligence. *Proc. IRE.* 49:8-30.   8

Minsky, M. (1965): Matter, mind and models. *In: Information Processing 1965.*   8
Proceedings of IFIP Congress 65, Vol. 1. (International Federation for
Information Processing, New York, May 24-29, 1965.) Kalenich, W.A., ed.
Washington, D.C.: Spartan Books, pp. 45-49.

Minsky, M. and Papert, P. (1972): Artificial intelligence progress report. Artificial   14
Intelligence Memorandum 252. Cambridge, Mass.: M.I.T. Artificial Intelligence
Laboratory.

Mitchell, D.E. and Blakemore, C. (1970): Binocular depth perception and the
corpus callosum. *Vision Res.* 10:49-54.

Morest, D.K. (1965): The laminar structure of the medial geniculate body of the   89
cat. *J. Anat.* 99:143-160.

Morest, D.K. (1971): Dendrodendritic synapses of cells that have axons: the fine   86,89
structure of the Golgi type II cell in the medial geniculate body of the cat.
Z. Anat. Entwicklungsgesch. 133:216-246.

Morrell, F. (1972): Integrative properties of parastriate neurons. *In: Brain and*   21
Human Behavior. Karczmar, A.G. and Eccles, J.C., eds. Berlin: Springer-Verlag,
pp. 259-289.

Mountcastle, V.B. (1957): Modality and topographic properties of single neurons of   45
cat's somatic sensory cortex. *J. Neurophysiol.* 20:408-434.

Mountcastle, V.B., Poggio, G.F., and Werner, G. (1963): The relation of thalamic
cell response to peripheral stimuli varied over an intensive continuum.
J. Neurophysiol. 26:807-834.

Movshon, J.A., Chambers, B.E.I., and Blakemore, C. (1972): Interocular transfer in
normal humans, and those who lack stereopsis. *Perception* 1:483-490.

Murphy, J.T., MacKay, W.A., and Johnson, F. (1973a): Differences between   162
cerebellar mossy and climbing fibre responses to natural stimulation of forelimb
muscle proprioceptors. *Brain Res.* 55:263-289.

Murphy, J.T., MacKay, W.A., and Johnson, F. (1973b): Responses of cerebellar   161
cortical neurons to dynamic proprioceptive inputs from forelimb muscles.
J. Neurophysiol. 36:711-723.

Murphy, J.T. and Sabah, N.H. (1970): The inhibitory effect of climbing fiber
activation on cerebellar Purkinje cells. *Brain Res.* 19:486-490.

Murphy, J.T. and Sabah, N.H. (1971): Cerebellar Purkinje cell responses to afferent
inputs. I. Climbing fiber activation. *Brain Res.* 25:449-467.

Murphy, J.T. and Sabah, N.H. (1971): Cerebellar Purkinje cell responses to afferent
inputs. II. Mossy fiber activation. *Brain Res.* 25:469-482.

Murphy, M.G. and O'Leary, J.L. (1971): Neurological deficit in cats with lesions of   133,164
the olivocerebellar system. *Arch. Neurol.* 24:145-157.

Murray, M.R. (1965): Nervous tissues *in vitro. In: Cells and Tissues in Culture.*   50
Methods, Biology and Physiology, Vol. 2. Willmer, E.N., ed. London: Academic
Press, pp. 373-455.

Nilsson, N.J. (1965): *Learning Machines. Foundations of Trainable Pattern-*   132
Classifying Systems. New York: McGraw-Hill.

Noda, H., Creutzfeldt, O.D., and Freeman, R.B., Jr. (1971): Binocular interaction
in the visual cortex of awake cats. *Exp. Brain Res.* 12:406-421.

Noda, H., Freeman, R.B., Jr., Gies, B., and Creutzfeldt, O.D. (1971): Neuronal
responses in the visual cortex of awake cats to stationary and moving targets.
Exp. Brain Res. 12:389-405.

Orlovskii, G.N. (1970a): Connexions of the reticulo-spinal neurones with the   158
"locomotor sections" of the brain stem. *Biophysics* 15:178-186.

Orlovskii, G.N. (1970b): Influence of the cerebellum on the reticulo-spinal   158
neurones during locomotion. *Biophysics* 15:928-936.

Orlovsky, G.N. (1972a): Activity of vestibulospinal neurons during locomotion.   158,164
Brain Res. 46:85-98.

Orlovsky, G.N. (1972b): The effect of different descending systems on flexor and   158,164
extensor activity during locomotion. *Brain Res.* 40:359-372.

Oscarsson, O. (1969): The sagittal organization of the cerebellar anterior lobe as   164
revealed by the projection patterns of the climbing fiber system. *In:*
Neurobiology of Cerebellar Evolution and Development. (Proceedings of the
First International Symposium of the Institute for Biomedical Research,
American Medical Association/Education and Research Foundation.) Llinás, R.,
ed. Chicago: American Medical Assoc., pp. 525-537.

Oscarsson, O. (1971): Recent developments on internal feedback. *Neurosciences*   92,148
Res. Prog. Bull. 9:98-103. Also *In: Neurosciences Research Symposium*
Summaries, Vol. 6. Schmitt, F.O. et al., eds. Cambridge, Mass.: M.I.T. Press,
1972, pp. 98-103.

Oscarsson, O. (1973): Functional organization of spinocerebellar paths. *In:*   91,93,
Handbook of Sensory Physiology, Vol. II. Somatosensory System. Iggo, A., ed.   148,149
Berlin: Springer-Verlag, pp. 339-380.

Oscarsson, O. and Rosén, I. (1966): Response characteristics of reticulocerebellar   93
neurones activated from spinal afferents. *Exp. Brain Res.* 1:320-328.

Oscarsson, O. and Uddenberg, N. (1964): Identification of a spinocerebellar tract   152
activated from forelimb afferents in the cat. *Acta Physiol. Scand.* 62:125-136.

Oscarsson, O. and Uddenberg, N. (1966): Somatotopic termination of spino-olivocerebellar path. *Brain Res.* 3:204-207.

Osen, K.K. (1969): Cytoarchitecture of the cochlear nuclei in the cat. *J. Comp.* 56
Neurol. 136:453-483.

Palkovits, M., Magyar, P., and Szentágothai, J. (1971a): Quantitative histological 66,79,
analysis of the cerebellar cortex in the cat. I. Number and arrangement in space 129
of the Purkinje cells. *Brain Res.* 32:1-13.

Palkovits, M., Magyar, P., and Szentágothai, J. (1971b): Quantitative histological 66,129
analysis of the cerebellar cortex in the cat. II. Cell numbers and densities in the
granular layer. *Brain Res.* 32:15-30.

Palkovits, M., Magyar, P., and Szentágothai, J. (1971c): Quantitative histological 66,67,68,
analysis of the cerebellar cortex in the cat. III. Structural organization of the 79,80,129,
molecular layer. *Brain Res.* 34:1-18. 152

Palkovits, M., Magyar, P., and Szentágothai, J. (1972): Quantitative histological 66,67,68,
analysis of the cerebellar cortex in the cat. IV. Mossy fiber-Purkinje cell 79,80,129,
numerical transfer. *Brain Res.* 45:15-29. 153,154

Pasik, P., Pasik, T., Hámori, J., and Szentágothai, J. (1973): Golgi type II 88
interneurons in the neuronal circuit of the monkey lateral geniculate nucleus.
Exp. Brain Res. 17:18-34.

Pecci Saavedra, J. and Vaccarezza, O.L. (1968): Synaptic organization of the 88
glomerular complexes in the lateral geniculate nucleus of *Cebus* monkey. *Brain
Res.* 8:389-393.

Pellionisz, A. (1970): Computer simulation of the pattern transfer of large 79
cerebellar neuronal fields. *Acta Biochim. Biophys. Acad. Sci. Hung.* 5:71-79.

Pellionisz, A. (1972): Computer simulation of the information preprocessing in the 79
input of the cerebellar cortex. *Acta Cybernetica* 3:157-169.

Pellionisz, A., Palkovits, M., Hámori, J., Pintér, E., and Szentágothai, J. (1974): 67
Quantitative comparison of the cerebellar synaptic organization of immobilized
and normal kittens. (Proceedings of the IV International Biophysical Congress,
Moscow, Aug., 1972.) (In press)

Pellionisz, A. and Szentágothai, J. (1973): Dynamic single unit simulation of a 79
realistic cerebellar network model. *Brain Res.* 49:83-99.

Pellionisz, A. and Szentágothai, J. (1974): Dynamic single unit simulation of a 79,129
realistic cerebellar network model. II. Purkinje cell activity within the basic
circuit and modified by inhibitory systems. *Brain Res.* 68:19-40.

Peters, A. and Palay, S.L. (1966): The morphology of laminae A and A_1 of the 86
dorsal nucleus of the lateral geniculate body of the cat. *J. Anat.* 100:451-486.

Peters, A. and Walsh, T.M. (1972): A study of the organization of apical dendrites 71,73,74
in the somatic sensory cortex of the rat. *J. Comp. Neurol.* 144:253-268.

Pettigrew, J.D. (1972a): The importance of early visual experience for neurons of 110,113
the developing geniculostriate system. *Invest. Ophthalmol.* 11:386-394.

Pettigrew, J.D. (1972b): The neurophysiology of binocular vision. *Sci. Am.*
227(2):84-95.

Pettigrew, J.D. (1973): Binocular neurones which signal change of disparity in   112
area 18 of cat visual cortex. *Nature New Biol.* 241:123-124.

Pettigrew, J.D. (1974a): The effect of selective visual experience on stimulus trigger   113
features of kitten cortical neurons. *Ann. N.Y. Acad. Sci.* 228:393-405.

Pettigrew, J.D. (1974b): The effect of visual experience on the development of   113
stimulus specificity by kitten cortical neurones. *J. Physiol.* 237:49-74.

Pettigrew, J.D., Nikara, T., and Bishop, P.O. (1968a): Binocular interaction on
single units in cat striate cortex: simultaneous stimulation by single moving slit
with receptive fields in correspondence. *Exp. Brain Res.* 6:391-410.

Pettigrew, J.D., Nikara, T., and Bishop, P.O. (1968b): Responses to moving slits by   22
single units in cat striate cortex. *Exp. Brain Res.* 6:373-390.

Poljakov, G.I. (1953): On the fine structure of the human cerebral cortex and   52
functional relations between its neurons. *Arkh. Anat. Gistol. Embriol.*
30(5):48-60.

Pompeiano, O. (1967): Functional organization of the cerebellar projections to the   158
spinal cord. *Prog. Brain Res.* 25:282-321.

Pöppel, E., Held, R.M., and Dowling, J.E. (1975): The visual field: psychophysics
and neurophysiology. *Neurosciences Res. Prog. Bull.* (In press)

Porter, B. (1969): *Synthesis of Dynamical Systems.* London: Nelson; New York: 36
Barnes and Noble, Inc.

Prigogine, I. (1947): *Étude Thermodynamique des Phénomènes Irreversibles.* Liège:
Desoer.

Rall, W. (1962): Electrophysiology of a dendritic neuron model. *Biophys. J.* 53,59,78
2(Suppl.):145-167.

Rall, W. (1964): Theoretical significance of dendritic trees for neuronal input- 53,54,55,
output relations. *In: Neural Theory and Modeling.* (Proceedings of the 1962   56,59,78
Ojai Symposium.) Reiss, R.F., ed. Stanford, Calif.: Stanford University Press,
pp. 73-97.

Rall, W. (1970): Dendritic neuron theory and dendrodendritic synapses in a simple
cortical system. *In: The Neurosciences: Second Study Program.* Schmitt, F.O.,
editor-in-chief. New York: Rockefeller University Press, pp. 552-565.

Rall, W., Shepherd, G.M., Reese, T.S., and Brightman, M.W. (1966): Dendrodendritic synaptic pathway for inhibition in the olfactory bulb. *Exp. Neurol.*
14:44-56.

Ramón-Moliner, E. (1962): An attempt at classifying nerve cells on the basis of   52
their dendritic patterns. *J. Comp. Neurol.* 119:211-227.

Ramón-Moliner, E. (1967): La différentiation morphologique des neurones. *Arch.* 48
Ital. Biol. 105:149-188.

Ramón-Moliner, E. (1968): The morphology of dendrites. *In: The Structure and* 48,156
Function of Nervous Tissue, Vol. I. Bourne, G.H., ed. New York: Academic
Press, pp. 205-267.

Ramón-Moliner, E. (1970): The structural and functional organization of the 48,74
neocortex. *Neurosciences Res. Prog. Bull.* 8:174-175. Also *In: Neurosciences
Research Symposium Summaries, Vol. 5.* Schmitt, F.O. et al., eds. Cambridge,
Mass.: M.I.T. Press, 1971, pp. 170-171.

Ramón-Moliner, E. and Nauta, W.J.H. (1966): The isodendritic core of the brain 43,46,47,
stem. *J. Comp. Neurol.* 126:311-335. 48,49,65,
106,156

Ramón y Cajal, S. (1899): Estudios sobra la cortezza cerebral humana. *Rev. Trim.* 73,108
Microscopia 4:1-63.

Ramón y Cajal, S. (1900): *Studien über die Hirnrinde des Menschen.* Leipzig: J.A.
Barth.

Ramón y Cajal, S. (1909): *Histologie du Système Nerveux de l'Homme et des* 16,43,58,
Vertébrés, Vol. 1. Paris: A. Maloine. (Reprinted in 1952 by Consejo Superior de 61,155
Investigaciones Cientificas, Instituto Ramón y Cajal, Madrid.)

Ramón y Cajal, S. (1911): *Histologie du Système Nerveux de l'Homme et des* 16,43,58,
Vertébrés, Vol. 2. Paris: A. Maloine. (Reprinted in 1955 by Consejo Superior de 65,98,95,
Investigaciones Cientificas, Instituto Ramón y Cajal, Madrid.) 98,154

Ramón y Cajal, S. (1935): Die Neuronenlehre. *In: Handbuch der Neurologie, Vol.* 59
I. Bumke, O. and Foerster, O., eds. Berlin: Springer-Verlag, pp. 887-994.

Ratliff, F. (1961): Inhibitory interaction and the detection and enhancement of 96
contours. *In: Sensory Communication.* (Contributions to the Symposium on
Principles of Sensory Communication, July 19-Aug. 1, 1959, Endicott House,
M.I.T.) Rosenblith, W.A., ed. Cambridge, Mass.: M.I.T. Press; New York: John
Wiley and Sons, Inc., pp. 183-203.

Reichardt, W. (1973): Musterinduzierte Flugorientierung. Verhaltens-Versuche an 29
der Fliege *Musca domestica. Naturwissenschaften* 60:122-138.

Reiss, R.F. (1964): A theory of resonant networks. *In: Neural Theory and* 43,84
Modeling. (Proceedings of the 1962 Ojai Symposium.) Reiss, R.F., ed. Stanford,
Calif.: Stanford University Press, pp. 105-137.

Réthelyi, M. and Szentágothai, J. (1973): Distribution and connections of afferent 62
fibres in the spinal cord. *In: Handbook of Sensory Physiology, Vol. II.
Somatosensory System.* Iggo, A. ed. Berlin: Springer-Verlag, pp. 207-252.

Rose, M. (1935): Anatomie des Grosshirns. (End-und Zwischenhirn.) *In: Handbuch* 44
der Neurologie, Vol. I. Bumke, O. and Foerster, O., eds. Berlin: Springer-Verlag,
pp. 541-587.

Rosén, I. and Asanuma, H. (1972): Peripheral afferent inputs to the forelimb area   98
of the monkey motor cortex: input-output relations. *Exp. Brain Res.*
14:257-273.

Rosenblatt, F. (1957): The perceptron: a perceiving and recognizing automaton.   132
Project PARA, Report 85-460-1. Ithaca, N.Y.: Cornell Aeronautical Laboratory.

Sabah, N. (1971): Reliability of computation in the cerebellum. *Biophys. J.*   142
11:429-445.

Sakmann, B. and Creutzfeldt, O.D. (1969): Scotopic and mesopic light adaptation
in the cat's retina. *Pflügers Arch.* 313:168-185.

Sanderson, K.J. (1971): Visual field projection columns and magnification factors   104
in the lateral geniculate nucleus of the cat. *Exp. Brain Res.* 13:159-177.

Sanderson, K.J., Bishop, P.O., and Darian-Smith, I. (1971): The properties of the
binocular receptive fields of lateral geniculate neurons. *Exp. Brain Res.*
13:178-207.

Sanides, F. (1970): Functional architecture of motor and sensory cortices in   18
primates in the light of a new concept of neocortex evolution. *In: The Primate
Brain.* (Advances in Primatology, Vol. 1.) Noback, C.R. and Montagna, W., eds.
New York: Appleton-Century-Crofts, Inc., pp. 137-208.

Scheibel, M.E. and Scheibel, A.B. (1955): The inferior olive. A Golgi study.   93
J. Comp. Neurol. 102:77-131.

Scheibel, M.E. and Scheibel, A.B. (1958): Structural substrates for integrative 43,49,59
patterns in the brain stem reticular core. *In: Reticular Formation of the Brain.*
(Henry Ford Hospital International Symposium, Detroit, Mich., Mar. 14-16,
1957.) Jasper, H.H., Proctor, L.D., Knighton, R.S., Noshay, W.C., and Costello,
R.T., eds. Boston, Mass.: Little, Brown and Co., pp. 31-68.

Scheibel, M.E. and Scheibel, A.B. (1966): Patterns of organization in specific and 43,88,89
nonspecific thalamic fields. *In: The Thalamus.* (Proceedings of the First
International Symposium sponsored by the Parkinson's Disease Information and
Research Center, College of Physicians and Surgeons, Columbia University.)
Purpura, D.P. and Yahr, M.D., eds. New York: Columbia University Press,
pp. 13-46.

Scheibel, M.E. and Scheibel, A.B. (1969): Terminal patterns in cat spinal cord. 43,53,59,
III. Primary afferent collaterals. *Brain Res.* 13:417-443.   60,64

Scheibel, M.E. and Scheibel, A.B. (1970): Elementary processes in selected   74
thalamic and cortical subsystems—the structural substrates. *In: The Neurosciences: Second Study Program.* Schmitt, F.O., editor-in-chief. New York:
Rockefeller University Press, pp. 443-457.

Schimert, J. (1939): Das Verhalten der Hinterwurzelkollateralen im Rückenmark.   61
Z. Anat. Entwicklungsgesch. 109:665-687.

Schweizer, H.-J. (1971): Experimentelle Untersuchungen über den Auge-Hand-Regelkreis bei der Durchführung einer Balancieraufgabe unter stroboskopischer Beleuchtung. *Kybernetik* 9:182-189.

Severin, F.V., Orlovskii, G.N., and Shik, M.L. (1968): Reciprocal influences on work of single motoneurons during controlled locomotion. *Bull. Exp. Biol. Med.* 66:713-716.   97

Shepherd, G.M. (1970): The olfactory bulb as a simple cortical system: experimental analysis and functional implications. *In: The Neurosciences: Second Study Program.* Schmitt, F.O., editor-in-chief, New York: Rockefeller University Press, pp. 539-552.   83

Sherrington, C.S. (1910): Flexion-reflex of the limb, crossed extension-reflex, and reflex stepping and standing. *J. Physiol.* 40:28-121.   164,165

Shik, M.L., Severin, F.V., and Orlovskii, G.N. (1966): Control of walking and running by means of electrical stimulation of the mid-brain. *Biophysics* 11:756-765.   158

Shkolnik-Yarros, E.G. (1963): Morphological data on the neuron connections in the cerebral cortex. *Gagr. Besedy* 4. (In Russian with English summary.)   52

Sholl, D.A. (1953): Dendritic organization in the neurons of the visual and motor cortices of the cat. *J. Anat.* 87:387-406.   48

Sholl, D.A. (1956): *The Organization of the Cerebral Cortex.* New York: John Wiley and Sons, Inc.   46,47,52

Sidman, R.L. (1974): Cell-cell recognition in the developing central nervous system. *In: The Neurosciences: Third Study Program.* Schmitt, F.O. and Worden, F.G., eds. Cambridge, Mass.: M.I.T. Press, pp. 743-758.   50

Sidman, R.L. and LaVail, J. (1974): Biology of the regenerating neuron. *Neurosciences Res. Prog. Bull.* (In press)

Simpson, J.I. and Alley, K.E. (1973): Trigger features for the visual climbing fiber input to rabbit vestibulo-cerebellum. *In: Program and Abstracts, Society for Neuroscience, Third Annual Meeting.* San Diego, Calif., p. 152.   140

Singer, W. and Creutzfeldt, O.D. (1970): Reciprocal lateral inhibition of on- and off-center neurones in the lateral geniculate body of the cat. *Exp. Brain Res.* 10:311-330.   104

Singer, W., and Pöppel, E., and Creutzfeldt, O. (1972): Inhibitory interaction in the cat's lateral geniculate nucleus. *Exp. Brain Res.* 14:210-226.   104

Smith, C.S. (1965): Structure, substructure, superstructure. *In: Structure in Art and in Science.* Kepes, G., ed. New York: George Braziller, Inc., pp. 29-41. Also *In: Rev. Mod. Physics* (1964): 36:524-532.

Smith, C.S. (1969): Structural hierarchy in inorganic systems. *In: Hierarchical Structures.* Whyte, L.L., Wilson, A., and Wilson, D., eds. New York: American Elsevier, pp. 61-85.

Snider, R.S. (1952): Interrelations of cerebellum and brain stem. *Res. Publ. Assoc.*   149
Res. Nerv. Ment. Dis. 30:267-281.

Sperry, R.W. (1950): Neural basis of the spontaneous optokinetic response   27,28,29
produced by visual inversion. *J. Comp. Physiol. Psychol.* 43:482-489.

Sperry, R.W. (1969): A modified concept of consciousness. *Psychol. Rev.*   11
76:532-536.

Sperry, R.W. (1974): Lateral specialization in the surgically separated hemispheres.   16
In: The Neurosciences: Third Study Program. Schmitt, F.O. and Worden, F.G.,
eds. Cambridge, Mass.: M.I.T. Press, pp. 5-19.

Spinelli, D.N. and Hirsch, H.V.B. (1971): Genesis of receptive field shapes in single   113
units of cat's visual cortex. *Fed. Proc.* 30:615. (Abstr.)

Spinelli, D.N., Hirsch, H.V.B., Phelps, R.W., and Metzler, J. (1972): Visual   114
experience as a determinant of the response characteristics of cortical receptive
fields in cats. *Exp. Brain Res.* 15:289-304.

Spinelli, D.N. and Metzler, J. (1975): The effect of restricted, prolonged visual   114
experience on the activity of single units in the visual cortex of adult cats. *Brain
Res.* (In press)

Spinelli, D.N., Metzler, J., and Phelps, R.W. (1973): Visual system in early and late   115
infancy. *In: Program and Abstracts, Society for Neuroscience, Third Annual
Meeting.* San Diego, Calif., p. 224.

Spoendlin, H. (1966): *The Organization of the Cochlear Receptor. Advances in*   83
Otolaryngology, Vol. 13. Basel: S. Karger.

Stone, J. and Hoffmann, K.P. (1972): Very slow-conducting ganglion cells in the   104
cat's retina: a major, new functional type? *Brain Res.* 43:610-616.

Straznicky, K. (1963): Function of heterotopic spinal cord segments investigated in   39
the chick. *Acta Biol. Acad. Sci. Hung.* 14:143-153.

Stryker, M. and Blakemore, C. (1972): Saccadic and disjunctive eye movements in
cats. *Vision Res.* 12:2005-2013.

Suga, N. (1969): Classification of inferior collicular neurones of bats in terms of   56
responses to pure tones, FM sounds and noise bursts. *J. Physiol.* 200:555-574.

Székely, G. (1965): Logical network for controlling limb movments in Urodela.
Acta Physiol. Acad. Sci. Hung. 27:285-289.

Székely, G. and Czéh, G. (1971a): Activity of spinal cord fragments and limbs   50,51,60
deplanted in the dorsal fin of urodele larvae. *Acta Physiol. Acad. Sci. Hung.*
40:303-312.

Székely, G. and Czéh, G. (1971b): Muscle activities of partially innervated limbs   50,51,60
during locomotion in Ambystoma. *Acta Physiol. Acad. Sci. Hung.* 40:269-286.

Page

Székely, G. and Szentágothai, J. (1962): Experiments with "model nervous   50,51
systems." *Acta Biol. Acad. Sci. Hung.* 12:253-269.

Szentágothai, J. (1943): Die zentrale Innervation der Augenbewegungen. *Arch.*   137
Psychiatr. Nervenkr. 116:721-760.

Szentágothai, J. (1950): The elementary vestibulo-ocular reflex arc. *J. Neuro-*   137
physiol. 13:395-407.

Szentágothai, J. (1951): Short propriospinal neurons and intrinsic connections of   61
the spinal gray matter. *Acta Morphol. Acad. Sci. Hung.* 1:81-94.

Szentágothai, J. (1952a): Kísérlet az idegrendszer szöveti elemeinek természetes   49
rendszerezésére. (An attempt at a "natural systematization" of nervous
elements.) *Magy. Tud. Akad., Biol. Orv. Tud. Osztl. Közl.* 3:365-412.

Szentágothai, J. (1952b): *Die Rolle der einzelnen Labyrinthrezeptoren bei der*   137
Orientation von Augen und Kopf im Raume. Budapest: Akadémiai Kiadó.

Szentágothai, J. (1961): Somatotopic arrangement of synapses of primary sensory   77
neurons in Clarke's column. *Acta Morphol. Acad. Sci. Hung.* 10:307-311.

Szentágothai, J. (1962): On the synaptology of the cerebral cortex. *In: Structure*   70
and Function of the Nervous System. Sarkisov, S.A., ed. Moscow: Medgiz,
pp. 6-14.

Szentágothai, J. (1963a): New data on the functional anatomy of synapses. *Magy.* 44,69,79
Tud. Akad., Biol. Orv. Tud. Osztl. Közl. 6:217-227.

Szentágothai, J. (1963b): The structure of the synapse in the lateral geniculate   86
body. *Acta Anat.* 55:166-185.

Szentágothai, J. (1964a): Anatomical aspects of junctional transformation. *In:*   43,86
Information Processing in the Nervous System, Vol. III. (Proceedings of the
International Union of Physiological Sciences, XXII International Congress,
Leiden, 1962.) Gerard, R.W. and Duyff, J.W., eds. Amsterdam: Excerpta Medica
Foundation, pp. 119-136.

Szentágothai, J. (1964b): Neuronal and synaptic arrangement in the substantia   43,52
gelatinosa Rolandi. *J. Comp. Neurol.* 122:219-239.

Szentágothai, J. (1964c): Propriospinal pathways and their synapses. *Prog. Brain*   43,61
Res. 11:155-177.

Szentágothai, J. (1965): The use of degeneration methods in the investigation of 43,44,69,
short neuronal connexions. *Prog. Brain Res.* 14:1-32.   70,79

Szentágothai, J. (1966): New anatomical concept of the brain stem. *In: Clinical*   49
Experiences in Brain Stem Disorders. (Conventus Neuropsychiatrici et EEG
Hungarici.) Juhász, P., Aszalós, Z., and Walsa, R. eds. Budapest: Ifjusági
Lapkiadó, pp. 15-28.

Szentágothai, J. (1967a): The anatomy of complex integrative units in the nervous   43,44,45,
system. *In: Recent Developments of Neurobiology in Hungary, Vol. 1. Results*   60,62,70,
in Neuroanatomy, Neurochemistry, Neuropharmacology and Neurophysiology.   72
Lissák, K., ed. Budapest: Akadémiai Kiadó, pp. 9-45.

Szentágothai, J. (1967b): Models of specific neuron arrays in thalamic relay nuclei.   43,49,88
Acta Morphol. Acad. Sci. Hung. 15:113-124.

Szentágothai, J. (1967c): Synaptic architecture of the spinal motoneuron pool. *In:*   61
Recent Advances in Clinical Neurophysiology, Electroencephalography and
Clinical Neurophysiology, Suppl. 25. (Proceedings of the Sixth International
Congress of Electroencephalography and Clinical Neurophysiology, Vienna,
Austria, Sept. 5-10, 1965.) Widén, L., ed. Amsterdam: Elsevier, pp. 4-19.

Szentágothai, J. (1968): Structuro-functional considerations of the cerebellar   49
neuron network. *Proc. IEEE* 56:960-968.

Szentágothai, J. (1969): Architecture of the cerebral cortex. *In: Basic Mechanisms*   44,49,70,
of the Epilepsies. Jasper, H.H., Ward, A.A., Jr., and Pope, A., eds. Boston: 71,72,79
Little, Brown and Co., pp. 13-28.

Szentágothai, J. (1970a): Les circuits neuronaux de l'écorce cérébrale. *Bull. Acad.*   71
R. Méd. Belg. 10:475-492.

Szentágothai, J. (1970b): Glomerular synapses, complex synaptic arrangements,   71,86,87,
and their operational significance. *In: The Neurosciences: Second Study*   88
Program. Schmitt, F.O., editor-in-chief. New York: Rockefeller University Press,
pp. 427-443.

Szentágothai, J. (1971): Some geometrical aspects of the neocortical neuropil. *Acta*   44,49,52,
Biol. Acad. Sci. Hung. 22:107-124.   73

Szentágothai, J. (1972a): The basic neuronal circuit of the neocortex. *In:*   44,71,72
Synchronization of EEG Activity in Epilepsies. (Symposium of the Austrian
Academy of Sciences, Vienna, Austria, Sept. 12-13, 1971.) Petsche, H. and
Brazier, M.A.B., eds. Vienna: Springer-Verlag, pp. 9-24.

Szentágothai, J. (1972b): Lateral geniculate body structure and eye movement.   74,89
Bibl. Ophthalmol. 82:178-188.

Szentágothai, J. (1973a): Synaptology of the visual cortex. *In: Handbook of*   71,73,79,
Sensory Physiology, Vol. VII/3. Part B. Central Processing of Visual Informa-   108
tion. Jung, R., ed., Berlin: Springer-Verlag, pp. 269-324.

Szentágothai, J. (1973b): Neuronal and synaptic architecture of the lateral
geniculate nucleus. *In: Handbook of Sensory Physiology, Vol. VII/3. Part B.*
Central Processing of Visual Information. Jung, R., ed. Berlin: Springer-Verlag,
pp. 141-176.

Szentágothai, J. (1974): From the last skirmishes around the neuron theory to the
functional anatomy of neuron networks. *In: The Neurosciences: Paths of*
Discovery. Worden, F.G., Swazey, J.P., and Adelman, G., eds. Cambridge, Mass.:
M.I.T. Press. (In press)

Szentágothai, J. and Albert, A. (1955): The synaptology of Clarke's column. *Acta 53,55,61, Morphol. Acad. Sci. Hung.* 5:43-51.   155

Szentágothai, J., Hámori, J., and Tömböl, T. (1966): Degeneration and electron   86 microscope analysis of the synaptic glomeruli in the lateral geniculate body. *Exp. Brain Res.* 2:283-301.

Szentágothai, J. and Pellionisz, A. (1971): The neuron network of the cerebellar cortex and attempt at its modelling by computer simulation. *In: First European Biophysics Congress, Vol. 5. Cells, Organs Including Nervous, Sensory, and Contractile Systems.* (Proceedings of Congress, Sept. 14-17, 1971, Baden, Austria.) Broda, E., Locker, A., and Springer-Lederer, H., eds. Vienna: Wiener Medizinischen Akademie, pp. 291-295.

Szentágothai, J. and Réthelyi, M. (1973): Cyto- and neuropil architecture of the   59,60 spinal cord. *In: New Developments in Electromyography and Clinical Neuro-physiology. Vol. 3, Human Reflexes, Pathophysiology of Motor Systems, Methodology of Human Reflexes.* Desmedt, J.E., ed. Basel: S. Karger, pp. 20-37.

Szentágothai, J. and Székely, G. (1956a): Elementary nervous mechanisms   28 underlying optokinetic responses, analyzed by contralateral eye grafts in urodele larvae. *Acta Physiol. Acad. Sci. Hung.* 10:43-55.

Szentágothai, J. and Székely, G. (1956b): Zum Problem der Kreuzung der   16 Nervenbahnen. *Acta Biol. Acad. Sci. Hung.* 6:215-229.

Teuber, H.-L. (1967): Lacunae and research approaches to them. I. *In: Brain   28 Mechanisms Underlying Speech and Language.* (Proceedings of a Conference held at Princeton, N.J., Nov. 9-12, 1965.) Darley, F.L., ed. New York: Grune and Stratton, Inc., pp. 204-216.

Thach, W.T. (1968): Discharge of Purkinje and cerebellar nuclear neurons during   164 rapidly alternating arm movements in the monkey. *J. Neurophysiol.* 31:785-797.

Tikhomirov, O.K. and Poznyanskaya, E.D. (1966-67): An investigation of visual   17 search as a means of analyzing heuristics. *Soviet Psychol.* 5:3-15.

Tömböl, T. (1967): Short neurons and their synaptic relations in the specific   89 thalamic nuclei. *Brain Res.* 3:307-326.

Tömböl, T. (1969a): Terminal arborizations in specific afferents in the specific thalamic nuclei. *Acta Morphol. Acad. Sci. Hung.* 17:273-284.

Tömböl, T. (1969b): Two types of short axon (Golgi 2nd) interneurons in the specific thalamic nuclei. *Acta Morphol. Acad. Sci. Hung.* 17:285-297.

Tsukahara, N. (1972): The properties of the cerebello-pontine reverberating circuit.   160 *Brain Res.* 40:67-71.

Uchizono, K. (1965): Characteristics of excitatory and inhibitory synapses in the central nervous system of the cat. *Nature* 207:642-643.

Page

Uchizono, K. (1967): Synaptic organization of the Purkinje cells in the cerebellum of the cat. *Exp. Brain Res.* 4:97-113.

Uttley, A.M. (1956): The probability of neural connexions. *Proc. Roy. Soc. B* 144:229-240.   46,49,52

Van der Loos, H. and Woolsey, T.A. (1973): Somatosensory cortex: structural alterations following early injury to sense organs. *Science* 179:395-398.   74,75

Van Essen, D. and Kelly, J. (1973): Correlation of cell shape and function in the visual cortex of the cat. *Nature* 241:403-405.   109

Vogt, O. (1903): Zur anatomischen Gliederung des Cortex cerebri. *J. Psychol. Neurol.* 2:160-180.   44

Vogt, C. and Vogt, O. (1919): Allgemeinere Ergebnisse unserer Hirnforschung. *J. Psychol. Neurol.* 25:279-462.   44

Von Békésy, G. (1967): *Sensory Inhibition.* Princeton, N.J.: Princeton University Press.

von Holst, E. and Mittelstaedt, H. (1950): Das Reafferenzprinzip. (Wechselwirkungen zwischen Zentralnervensystem und Peripherie.) *Naturwissenschaften* 37:464-476.   27,28,29

Voogd, J. (1964): *The Cerebellum of the Cat. Structure and Fibre Connexions.* Philadelphia: F.A. Davis Co.   152

Voogd, J. (1967): Comparative aspects of the structure and fibre connexions of the mammalian cerebellum. *Prog. Brain Res.* 25:94-134.   150

Voogd, J. (1969): The importance of fiber connections in the comparative anatomy of the mammalian cerebellum. *In: Neurobiology of Cerebellar Evolution and Development.* (Proceedings of the First International Symposium of the Institute for Biomedical Research, American Medical Association/Education and Research Foundation.) Llinás, R., ed. Chicago: American Medical Assoc., pp. 493-514.   148,152, 162,164

Wässle, H. and Creutzfeldt, O.D. (1973): Spatial resolution in visual system: a theoretical and experimental study on single units in the cat's lateral geniculate body. *J. Neurophysiol.* 36:13-27.   124

Weiskrantz, L. (1972): Behavioural analysis of the monkey's visual nervous system. *Proc. Roy. Soc. B* 182:427-455.   21

Weiss, P. (1936): A study of motor coordination and tonus in deafferented limbs of Amphibia. *Am. J. Physiol.* 115:461-475.

Weiss, P. (1950a): The deplantation of fragments of nervous system in amphibians. I. Central reorganization and the formation of nerves. *J. Exp. Zool.* 113:397-461.   50,51,63

Weiss, P. (1950b): An introduction to genetic neurology. *In: Genetic Neurology.*   16,39,59
*Problems of the Development, Growth, and Regeneration of the Nervous
System and of Its Functions.* (Conference sponsored by the International Union
of Biological Sciences subsidized by UNESCO.) Weiss, P. ed. Chicago: University
·of Chicago Press, pp. 1-39.

Werner, G. (1970): The topology of the body representation in the somatic afferent   15
pathway. *In: The Neurosciences: Second Study Program.* Schmitt, F.O.,
editor-in-chief. New York: Rockefeller University Press, pp. 605-617.

Werner, G. (1972): Somatotopic projections. *Neurosciences Res. Prog. Bull.*   19
10:262-268. Also *In: Neurosciences Research Symposium Summaries, Vol. 7.*
Schmitt, F.O. et al, eds. Cambridge, Mass.: M.I.T. Press, 1973, pp. 262-268.

Werner, G. (1974): Neural information processing with stimulus feature extractors.   21
In: The Neurosciences: Third Study Program. Schmitt, F.O. and Worden, F.G.,
eds. Cambridge, Mass.: M.I.T. Press, pp. 171-183.

Werner, G. and Whitsel, B.L. (1968): Topology of the body representation in   19
somatosensory area I of primates. *J. Neurophysiol.* 31:856-869.

Werner, G. and Whitsel, B.L. (1973): Functional organization of the somatosensory
cortex. *In: Handbook of Sensory Physiology, Vol. II. Somatosensory System.*
Iggo, A., ed. Berlin: Springer-Verlag, pp. 621-700.

Whitaker, H.P. (1962): Design capabilities of model reference adaptive systems.   36
Report R-374. Cambridge, Mass.: M.I.T. Instrumentation Laboratory.

Whitaker, H.P. (1963): Use of model-reference adaptive control to achieve a   36
specified performance. Report R-407. Cambridge, Mass.: M.I.T. Instrumentation
Laboratory.

Whitsel, B.L., Petrucelli, L.M., and Werner, G. (1969): Symmetry and connectivity   18
in the map of the body surface in somatosensory area II of primates.
J. Neurophysiol. 32:170-183.

Whitsel, B.L., Roppolo, J.R., and Werner, G. (1972): Cortical information   20,22,56,
processing of stimulus motion on primate skin. *J. Neurophysiol.* 35:691-717.   98

Wilson, H.R. and Cowan, J.D. (1972): Excitatory and inhibitory interactions in 43,51,117,
localized populations of model neurons. *Biophys. J.* 12:1-24.   124

Wilson, H.R. and Cowan, J.D. (1973): A mathematical theory of the functional
dynamics of cortical and thalamic nervous tissue. *Kybernetik* 13:55-80.

Wilson, V.J. and Burgess, P.R. (1962): Disinhibition in the cat spinal cord.   96
J. Neurophysiol. 25:392-404.

Wilson, V.J., Talbot, W.H., and Kato, M. (1964): Inhibitory convergence upon   96
Renshaw cells. *J. Neurophysiol.* 27:1063-1079.

Winograd, S. and Cowan, J.D. (1963): *Reliable Computation in the Presence of*   132,142
Noise. Cambridge, Mass.: M.I.T. Press.

Woolsey, C.N. (1958): Organization of somatic sensory and motor areas of the   18
cerebral cortex. *In: Biological and Biochemical Bases of Behavior.* Harlow, H.F.
and Woolsey, C.N., eds. Madison, Wis.: University of Wisconsin Press, pp. 63-81.

Woolsey, C.N. and Fairman, D. (1946): Contralateral, ipsilateral, and bilateral   18
representation of cutaneous receptors in somatic areas I and II of the cerebral
cortex of pig, sheep, and other mammals. *Surgery* 19:684-702.

Woolsey, C.N., Marshall, W.H., and Bard, P. (1942): Representation of cutaneous   18
tactile sensibility in the cerebral cortex of the monkey as indicated by evoked
potentials. *Bull. Johns Hopkins Hosp.* 70:399-441.

Woolsey, T.A. and Van der Loos, H. (1970): The structural organization of layer IV 45,74,75
in the somatosensory region (S I) of mouse cerebral cortex. The description of a
cortical field composed of discrete cytoarchitectonic units. *Brain Res.*
17:205-242.

Wyburn, G.M., Pickford, R.W., and Hirst, R.J. (1964): *Human Senses and*   101
Perception. Edinburgh: Oliver and Boyd.

Young, J.Z. (1964): *A Model of the Brain.* Oxford: Oxford University Press.   8,10,16

INDEX

Abbreviations, 166
Activation, of function generator, 34
  in theory of tasks, 34
  see also Feedback; Feedforward
Active touch, and somatosensory cortex, 18-20
Afferent systems, organization principles,
  81-90
Aizerman, M.A., cit., 146
Albert, A., cit., 53, 55, 61, 155
Albus, K., cit., 105
Alley, K.E., cit., 140
Allodendritic nerve cells, 47-49
Ambiguity of disparity, in stereograms, 121
Ambiguous figures, girl-crone, 99-100
  Dalmatian dog, 99
  Necker cube, 100
  vase-two faces, 101
Analysis-by-synthesis view of perception, 10
Andersen, P., cit., 88, 96, 119
Andreeva, E.A., cit., 146
Anninos, P.A., cit., 51
Arbib, M.A., 1-198, 28,105,134; cit., 8, 9,
  23, 24, 26, 38, 40, 121, 123, 159,
  161, 163
Armstrong, D.M., cit., 147, 162
Arshavsky, Y.I., cit., 148, 165
Asanuma, H., cit., 98
Atwood, R.P., cit., 130
Auditory system, neuron couplings, 82-90

Ballistic movements of limbs, 130-131
Ball-park mechanism, 34-35
  in theory of tasks, 36, 38
Barlow, H.B., 117; cit., 85
Barrel structure, cortical, in mouse vibrissae
  system, 22, 74-76
Basic cerebellar circuit, 160
Basket cells, 72
Bell, C.C., cit., 162
Benevento, L.A., 107; cit., 105, 108
Bernstein, N., 33, 57; cit., 157
Beurle, R.L., cit., 43, 117
Blakemore, C., vi, 105, 108, 111, 112, 113,
  114, 117; cit., 22, 105, 108, 112,
  113, 114
Bobrow, L., cit., 40
Bodian, D., cit., 49
Body topography in SI, 19
Boring, E.G., 100

Boylls, C.C., vi, 6, 35, 133, 139, 140, 158-
  165; cit., 138, 139, 158
Boylls's synergy controller model, 35, 158,
  159, 165
Braitenberg, V., vi, 5, 29, 31, 130-131, 152;
  cit., 16, 130
Braitenberg's timing model of cerebellum, 130-
  131, 132
Brodal, A., 45, 153, 160
Brooks, V.B., cit., 96
Brown, J.E., cit., 104
Bullock, T.H., cit., 39, 43
Bunge, M.B., cit., 50
Bunge, R.P., cit., 50
Burchfiel, J.L., cit., 20, 21
Burgess, P.R., cit., 96
Burns, B.D., cit., 112, 120

Camera lucida principle of neural connections,
  16
Carraher, R.G., cit., 99
Cartridges (apical dendrites), 72
Cellules à double bouquet, 72
Cerebellum, computer simulation, 162-163
  cortex, basic circuitry, 125-133
    neuron network, 78
  function, and synergies, 157-165
  impulse transmission to and from, spatio-
    temporal plot, 145
  modules, 65-69
  in motor control, feedback and feedforward,
    133-140
    function, 5-6, 125-165
  projections, 147-157
  relay systems, 155-157
  in spinal control of limb movement, 140-
    141
Cerebral modules, 70-74
Cerebrocerebellar interactions, 140-146
Chandelier cells, 71-72
Chernov, V.I., cit., 146
Chow, K.L., cit., 74
Cleland, B.G., cit., 104
Climbing fibers, in basic cerebellar cir-
    cuit, 160-161
  in cerebellar motor control, 138-140
  in computer simulation of cerebellum,
    162-165
Codon, in cerebellum, 132

Colonnier, M., cit., 70, 73, 86
Co-moving sets, 26
Comparator loop, of motor system, 91-95
Computer simulation of cerebellum model, 162-163
Connectivity, in cerebellar cortex, 65-69
    specific, modules of, 69-74
    see also Synapses
Cooke, J.D., cit., 147
Cooper, G.F., cit., 114
Cooperative phenomena, in stereopsis, 99, 103
Coordinated movement, minimal structural requirements, 39-40
Corollary discharge, 27-29
    structural basis, 97
Cortex, stereopsis neurophysiology, 104-115
Cortical barrels (organs), 22, 45, 74-76
Cortical connections, in areas of vision and touch, 20-23
Cortical mapping, 19-23
Corticonuclear projection, 153
Cosgriff, R.L., cit., 146
Cowan, J.D., vi, 5, 117, 118, 120, 132-133; cit., 43, 51, 117, 124, 132, 142
Cragg, B.G., cit., 99
Craik, K.J.W., cit., 8
Crain, S.M., cit., 50
Creutzfeldt, O.D., vi, 88, 105-109, 111, 113; cit., 14, 29, 57, 104, 111, 124
Creutzfeldt model, 105-107, 108
Crossing of neural pathways, 15-16
Cuneocerebellar projection, 150-151
Cyclopean perception, 101
Czéh, G., 63; cit., 50, 51, 60, 63

Dalmatian dog ambiguous figure, 99
Dendritic arborization, 156
    classification, 46-50
Dendritic geometry model of Rall, 53-56
Dendritic orientation to axonal arborization, 52-53
Deplantation studies, 50-52, 63-64
Dertouzos, M.L., cit., 33
Dev, P., vi, 5, 110, 121, 123; cit., 117
Dev's model of figure-ground separation, 117, 120-124
Didday, R.L., cit., 23, 24, 26, 27
Dipole-array model of stereopsis, 115-117
Disparity array, 121-123
Disparity-tuned neurons, 109-113
Dressler, R.M., cit., 36

Dreyer, D.A., cit., 19
Dubner, R., cit., 21
Duffy, F.H., cit., 20, 21

Eccles, J.C., vi, 5, 129, 140-143; cit., 44, 54, 65, 66, 69, 70, 88, 96, 119, 127, 128, 131, 141, 142, 143, 144, 145, 146, 149, 151, 154, 156
Economo, C.F. von, cit., 44
Edds, M.V., Jr., vi
Ekerot, C.-F., cit., 148, 149, 150, 151
Environment, interaction with, general principles, 7-16
Erulkar, S.D., cit., 56, 85
Evans, E.F., cit., 21, 22
Evarts, E.V., cit., 11, 27, 29, 37, 38, 91, 98, 148
Evolving movement, 143-144
Excitation, distribution in modular spatial patterns, 69-74
Eye movements, and visual perception, 23-27

Fairman, D., cit., 18
Famiglietti, E.V., Jr., cit., 86, 88
Farley, B.G., cit., 43
Feature detectors, 23, 81
Feature extraction, 56, 81, 85
Feedback, in cerebellar control, 133-140
    inhibition of, in cerebellar circuitry, 126
    internal loops, organization principles, 91-98
    in motor control, 33-39
        large-scale, organization, 91-95
        local recurrent couplings, 95-97
        spinal, 37-39
        structural basis of corollary discharge, 97
        types, 91
Feedforward, in cerebellar control, 133-140
    inhibition of, in cerebellar circuitry, 126
    in motor control, 33-39
Fender, D., cit., 103, 120
Figure-ground reversal, 100-101
Figure-ground separation model of stereopsis, 5, 110, 120-124
Flocculus, in cerebellar motor control, 134-140
Fly, optomotor behavior, 29-32

Foreground-background reference, 31
Forssberg, H., cit., 158
Foveal slide generator, 24
Foveation, 23
Fox, C.A., cit., 126
Freeman, J.A., cit., 130
Frequency modulation recognition, 85
Frisby, J.P., vi
Frog tectum model, 26
Function generator, activation of, in Greene's
    theory of tasks, 34, 165
    role in cerebellar function, 157-158,
    165
Functional amputation, 71-73
Fuster, J.M., cit., 104

Gazzaniga, M.S., cit., 16
Gelfand, I.M., 157; cit., 35, 157
Gerlach, J., cit., 42
Gibson, J.J., cit., 18
Girl-crone ambiguous figure, 99-100
Globus, A., cit., 58, 74, 79
Gonshor, A., cit., 135, 140
Götz, K.G., cit., 29
Graham, D., cit., 146
Graham, H.L., cit., 33
Granit, R., cit., 126, 162
Gratings, 109
Greene, P.H., vi, 34, 37, 40, 146, 157, 165;
    cit., 33, 34, 62, 146
Greene's theory of tasks, 34-35
Gregory, R.L., cit., 8
Grillner, S., cit., 158, 164
Guillery, R.W., cit., 58, 86
Gurfinkel, V.S., cit., 146

Hajdu, F., cit., 87
Hámori, J., 86; cit., 52, 68, 89
Harrison, J.M., cit., 56, 57
Harth, E.M., cit., 51
Hartline, H.K., cit., 96
Hebb, D., cit., 113
Helmholtz, H., cit., 27
Henneman, E., cit., 53, 59
Heterarchy, in artificial intelligence, 14
Hierarchy, of anatomical structures, 13-14, 40
    of levels of description, 13
    of motor control, 32-40
    of nervous system organization, 1, 10-14,
    76-80
    of visual cortical neurons, 111-113

Hillman, D.E., cit., 71
Hirsch, H.V.B., cit., 113
Hoffmann, K.P., cit., 104
Holmes, G., cit., 125
Homsy, Y.M., 1-198
Horridge, G.A., cit., 43
Hubel, D.H., 72; cit., 21, 22, 45, 105, 106,
    109, 111, 112
Hultborn, H., cit., 96, 97
Hypothesis-confirmation map, 25, 27
Hysteresis, 99-100, 103
    theories, 115-124

Idiodendritic nerve cells, 47-49, 65
Inactivation response, of Purkinje cells, in
    computer simulation of cerebellum,
    162
Ingle, D., cit., 80
Inhibition, distribution in modular spatial
    patterns, 69-74
Inhibitory interneurons, 44
Input-output relations of cerebellar projec-
    tions, 153-155
Integrative units of neural tissue, 45
Internal feedback, 38, 91-98
    see also Feedback
Internal model of world, role of memory, 8-10
Intersegmental reflexes, 38
Intrasegmental reflexes, 37
Irving, R., cit., 56, 57
Isodendritic nerve cells, 46-49, 65
Ito, M., 5, 134-139; cit., 36, 133, 134, 135,
    136, 137, 138, 140

Jansen, J., cit., 153
Jones, E.G., cit., 20
Julesz, B., vi, 5, 100, 111, 117, 120-123, 133;
    cit., 101, 102, 103, 115, 116, 120,
    133
Jung, R., cit., 109

Katchalsky, A. Katzir, cit., 119
Kauffman, S., cit., 51
Kawasaki, T., cit., 162
Kelly, J., cit., 109
Kilmer, W.L., cit., 49
"Knowledge of results" feedback in motor con-
    trol, 91
Kornhuber, H.H., cit., 130

Koskinas, G.N., cit., 44
Kots, Y.N., cit., 164
Dropfl, W.J., cit., 133
Kuhnt, U., 107

Land, M.F., cit., 80
Larson, B., vi, 148-152; cit., 148, 149, 150, 152
Layer-by-layer analysis of neuron networks, 76-80
Lázár, G., cit., 57
Learning model of cerebellum, 131-133
Least interaction principle, definition, 35
Legéndy, C.R., cit., 51
Leicht, R., cit., 149
Leiman, A.L., cit., 74
Leontovich, T.A., cit., 49
Lettvin, J.Y., cit., 77
Le Vay, S., cit., 88
Levick, W.R., cit., 85, 104
Limb movement, control, 140-141
   patterns, 39
Lindström, S., cit., 148
Line detectors in cat visual system, 111-113
Linearizing control, 146
Llinás, R., cit., 70, 71, 93, 128, 156, 160
Local feature map, 25
Loeb, J.M., cit., 146
Long-term memory, in internal model of world, 9-10
Lorente de Nó, R., cit., 43, 44, 79, 95, 108, 135
Lotka-Volterra equations, 119
Lundberg, A., 96; cit., 97, 148

MacColl, L.A., cit., 146
McCulloch, W.S., cit., 14
MacKay, D.M., vi, 26, 106; cit., 8, 28
McRuer, D.T., cit., 146
Maekawa, K., cit., 136, 137, 140
Magnus, R., 164
Major, D., cit., 104
Majorossy, K., cit., 89
Malsburg, C. von der, cit., 113, 124
Mannen, H., cit., 61, 155
Marin-Padilla, M., cit., 70
Marr, D., 5, 131-133, 134; cit., 117, 131, 135
Marr's learning model of cerebellum, 131-133

Master neurons, 39
Maturana, H.R., cit., 57
Melvill Jones, G., cit., 135, 140
Memory, long- and short-term, 9-10
Mendell, L.M., cit., 53, 59
Merton, P.A., cit., 146
Mesencephalic locomotion, cerebellar function in, 158-165
Metzler, J., cit., 114
Milner, B., cit., 16
Minsky, M., cit., 8, 14
Mitchell, D.E., cit., 114
Mittelstaedt, H., 26; cit., 27, 28, 29
Model-reference control, 36
Modules, cerebellar, 65-69
   cerebral, 70-74
   large-scale organoid, 74-76
   in neuropil organization, 58-80
   of specific connectivity, 69-74
Morest, D.K., cit., 86, 89
Morrell, F., cit., 21
Mossy fiber action, in cerebellar cortex, 128-130
Motion detectors, see Movement detectors
Motor control, cerebellar function, 5-6, 125-165
   complexity and hierarchies, 40-41
   hierarchies, 32-41
   internal feedback loops, organization principles, 91-98
Mountcastle, V.B., cit., 45
Movement, coordinated, minimal structural requirements, 39-40
   detectors, 22, 30-32
Multiple representations of sensory inputs, 17-32
Multiplicity of connections, 95
Murphy, J.T., cit., 161, 162
Murphy, M.G., cit., 133, 164
Murray, M.R., cit., 50

Natsui, T., cit., 137, 140
Nauta, W.J.H., 136; cit., 43, 46, 47, 48, 49, 65, 106, 156
Necker cube, 99-100
Neocortex, modular system, 70-74
Neural arborization, 42-58, 89, 156
   see also Neuron
Neurl networks, concepts, 52-58
   Reiss, 43, 84
   Wilson-Cowan model, 43, 51, 117-120, 124
   see also Neuron

Neuron, coupling, in sensory systems, 82-90
    machine, 44, 69
    networks, 42-58
        layer-by-layer analysis, 76-80
    pathways, crossing, 15-16
Neuropil, 45
    modular structure, 58-80
    stacked chips, 58-65
Nilsson, N.J., 132

Oculomotor control, cerebellar, 133-140
O'Leary, J.L., cit., 133, 164
Olfactory system, neuron couplings, 82-90
Onesto, N., cit., 130
Optomotor behavior in the fly, 29-32
Order-disorder transitions, 99, 117
Orlovsky, G.N., cit., 158, 164
Oscarsson, O., cit., 91, 92, 93, 148, 149, 152, 164
Osen, K.K., cit., 56
Output feature clusters (OFC's), 24-27, 35

Palay, S.L., cit., 86
Palkovits, M., cit., 66, 67, 68, 79, 80, 127, 129, 152, 153, 154
Papert, P., cit., 14
Parallel fibers, synaptic contacts with Purkinje cells, 66-69
Parallel inhibition, 96
Pasik, P., 86; cit., 88
Pasik, T., 86
Pecci Saavedra, J., cit., 88
Pellionisz, A., cit., 67, 79, 129
Perception, analysis-by-synthesis view, 10
    slide box and slide file metaphors, 9-10
    stereopsis, 99-103
Perceptron scheme, 132
Perceptual transition from order to disorder, 99
Peters, A., cit., 71, 73, 74, 86, 88
Pettigrew, J.D., vii, 100, 109, 117; cit., 22 110, 112, 113
Pettigrew's model, 109-111
Phillips, C.G., cit., 126, 162
Pinhole camera principle of neural connections, 16
Poker chip model of the neuropil, 49
Poljakov, G.I., cit., 52
Pompeiano, O., cit., 158

Porter, B., cit., 36
Positive feedback, cerebellar, 159-163
Postcentral tactile (SI) area, 18-20
Potential command, 7-8
Powell, T.P.S., cit., 20
Poznyanskaya, E.D., cit., 17
Precentral motor (MI) area, 18
Purkinje cells, modular arrangement, 65-69

Rall, W., cit., 53, 54, 55, 56, 78
Ramón y Cajal, S., 72; cit., 16, 43, 58, 59, 61, 65, 73, 89, 98, 108, 154, 155
Ramón-Moliner, E., vii, 153, 157; cit., 43, 46, 47, 48, 49, 52, 65, 74, 106, 156
Random-dot stereograms, 100-103, 109-111, 120-123
Ratliff, F., cit., 96
Reafference principle, 26, 28-29
Recurrent inhibition, 96
Recurrent local neuron couplings, 95-97
Redundancy of potential command, 7-8, 26
Reichardt, W., cit., 29
Reiss, R.F., cit., 43, 84
Relay nuclei, sensory, 84-90
Renshaw cell recurrent coupling, 96-97
Representations, multiple, 17-32
Response feedback in motor control, 91
Réthelyi, M., cit., 59, 60, 62, 87
Reticulocerebellar reverberatory loop, 159-160
Retinal ganglion cells, 104
Reverberating circuits, see Recurrent local neuron couplings
Reverberatory loop, cerebellar, 159-163
Reversal in ambiguous figures, 99-100
Rope ladder phenomenon in spiny dendrites, 52
Rose, M., cit., 44
Rosén, I., cit., 93, 98
Rosenblatt, F., cit., 132

Sabah, N., cit., 142, 162
Sanderson, K.J., cit., 104
Sanides, F., cit., 18
Scheibel, A.B., cit., 43, 49, 53, 58, 59, 60, 64, 74, 79, 88, 89, 93
Scheibel, M.E., cit., 43, 49, 53, 59, 60, 64, 74, 88, 89, 93
Schimert, J., cit., 61
Schmitt, F.O., vii

Second sensory (SII) area, 18
Self-reexciting chain, *see* Recurrent local
    neuron couplings
Semantic feedback, 111
Sensory systems, neuronal and synaptic organ-
    izations, 82-90
Severin, F.V., cit., 97
Shepherd, G.M., cit., 82, 83
Sherrington, C.S., 164, 165
Shik, M.L., cit., 158
Shkolnik-Yarros, E.G., cit., 52
Sholl, D.A., cit., 46, 47, 48, 52
Short-term memory, in internal model of world,
    9-10
Sidman, R.L., cit., 50
Simpson, J.I., cit., 136-140
Singer, W., cit., 104
Slide box metaphor of perception, 9-10, 24-
    26
Slide file metaphor of perception, 9-10
Smith, C.S., vii
Snider, R.S., cit., 147
Somatosensory cortex, modular structure, 74-
    76
Somatosensory system, 17-23
    neuron couplings, 83-90
Somatotopy, of nervous system, 14-16
Specific neuron machine, 44
Sperry, R.W., cit., 11, 16, 27, 28, 29
Spinal control of movement, 37-39
Spinelli, D.N., cit., 113, 114, 115
Spinocerebellar projections, 147-153
Spoendlin, H., cit., 83
Sprague, J.M., cit., 80
Stacked chips of neuropil, 58-65
Stellate nerve cells, 46-49
Stereopsis, 4-5
    cortical neurophysiology, 104-115
    integrating theories, 115-124
    perceptual level, 99-103
Stone, J., cit., 104
Straznicky, K., cit., 39
Structural organization, requirements for
    control systems, 42
Subcortical sensory relay nuclei, 84-90
Suga, H, cit., 56
Superior colliculus, collicular pathways, 23-
    27
    spatial arrays, 25-27
Supplementary motor (MII) area, 18
Synapses, in cerebellar cortex, 65-69
    crossing over and parallel, 52-53

Synapses *(continued)*
    in sensory systems, organization, 82-90
    see also Connectivity
Synergy, 6
    and cerebellar function, 157-165
    controller model, 159-165
Syrovegin, A.V., cit., 164
Székely, G., 16, 28, 51, 63; cit., 16, 28,
    50, 51, 57, 60, 63
Szentágothai, J., 1-198, 16, 28, 45, 51, 54,
    66, 78, 82-83, 86, 90, 94-95, 105,
    134, 152, 162; cit., 16, 28, 43, 44,
    45, 49, 50, 51, 52, 53, 55, 59, 60,
    61, 62, 69, 70, 71, 72, 73, 74, 77,
    79, 86, 87, 88, 89, 108, 129, 137,
    155
Szikla, G., cit., 160

Temperley, H.N.V., cit., 99
Teuber, H.-L., cit., 28
Thach, W.T., cit., 164
Thurston, J.B., cit., 99
Tight input-output couplings, 97-98
Tikhomirov, O.K., cit., 17
Timing model of cerebellum, 130-131
Tissue cultures, in neural network study, 50-
    52
Tobin, E.A., cit., 105, 108, 112
Tömböl, T., cit., 89
Touch, active, 18-20
    see also Somatosensory system
Triadic coupling of subcortical sensory relay
    nuclei, 86-88
Tsetlin, M.L., 157
Tsukahara, N., cit., 160
Tuning action, in Greene's theory of tasks,
    34-35
Tuning inputs, role in generation of patterns,
    33-36
Two-field model of stereopsis, 5, 117-120

Uddenberg, N., cit., 152
"die Umkehr," 164
Unique neurons, 39
Uttley, A.M., cit., 46, 49, 52

Vaccarezza, O.L., cit., 88
Van der Loos, H., vii, 22, 74, 153; cit., 45,
    74, 75
Van Essen, D., cit., 109

Vase-two faces figure, ambiguity, 100-101
Vestibuloocular reflex (VOR), 133-140
Vestibulospinal reflex (VSR), 133-136
Vision, cortical sensory system compared with
    somatosensory system, 20-23
Visual cortex, circuitry development, 113-115
    see also Stereopsis
Visual cortical neurons, hierarchy, 111-113
Visual display system, of Dertouzos, 33-34
Visual perception and eye movements, 23-27
Visual system, neuron couplings, 82-90
Vogt, C., cit., 44
Vogt, O., cit., 44
von Holst, E., 28, 97; cit., 27, 28, 29
Voogd, J., cit., 148, 150, 152, 162, 164
Vordergrund-Hintergrund-Beziehung, 31

W cells, 104
Walsh, T.M., cit., 71, 73, 74
Wässle, H., cit., 124
Weiskrantz, L., cit., 21
Weiss, P., 50; cit., 16, 39, 50, 51, 53
Werner, G., vii; cit., 15, 19, 21
Whiskers, receptors in somatosensory cortex,
    modular structure, 74-76

Whitaker, H.P., cit., 36
Whitsel, B.L., cit., 18, 20, 22, 56, 98
Wiesel, T.N., 72; cit., 21, 22, 45, 105,
    106, 109, 111, 112
Wilson, H.R., 5, 120; cit., 43, 51, 117, 124
Wilson, V.J., cit., 96
Wilson-Cowan model, 43, 51, 80, 117-120, 124
Wing movement patterns, 39
Winograd, S., cit., 132, 142
Winograd-Cowan model of reliable computation
    in presence of noise, 132-133
Woolsey, C.N., 18; cit., 18
Woolsey, T.A., 74; cit., 45, 74, 75
Worden, F.G., vii
Wyburn, G.M., cit., 101

X cells, 104

Y cells, 104
Young, J.Z., cit., 8, 10, 16

Zeevi, Y.Y., vii;
Zeki, S.M., cit., 21
Zhukova, G.P., cit., 49

DATE DUE